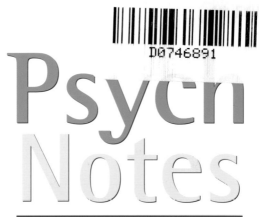

D0746891

Psych
Notes

Clinical Pocket Guide

Darlene D. Pedersen, MSN, APRN, PMHCNS

Purchase additional copies of this book at your health science bookstore or directly from F. A. Davis by shopping online at www.fadavis.com or by calling 800-323-3555 (US) or 800-665-1148 (CAN)

A Davis's Notes Book

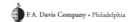

F.A. Davis Company • Philadelphia

F. A. Davis Company
1915 Arch Street
Philadelphia, PA 19103
www.fadavis.com

Printed in China

Last digit indicates print number: 10 9 8 7 6 5 4 3 2 1

Publisher, Nursing: Robert G. Martone

Manager, Freelance Development: William F. Welsh

Assistant Project Editor: Christina Snyder

Design and Illustration Manager: Carolyn O'Brien

As new scientific information becomes available through basic and clinical research, recommended treatments and drug therapies undergo changes. The author(s) and publisher have done everything possible to make this book accurate, up to date, and in accord with accepted standards at the time of publication. The author(s), editors, and publisher are not responsible for errors or omissions or for consequences from application of the book, and make no warranty, expressed or implied, in regard to the contents of the book. Any practice described in this book should be applied by the reader in accordance with professional standards of care used in regard to the unique circumstances that may apply in each situation. The reader is advised always to check product information (package inserts) for changes and new information regarding dose and contraindications before administering any drug. Caution is especially urged when using new or infrequently ordered drugs.

Place 2⅞ × 2⅞ **Sticky Notes** here
for a convenient and refillable note pad

✓**HIPAA compliant**
✓**OSHA compliant**

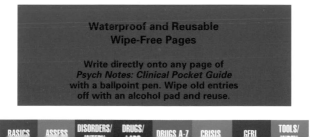

Waterproof and Reusable
Wipe-Free Pages

Write directly onto any page of
Psych Notes: Clinical Pocket Guide
with a ballpoint pen. Wipe old entries
off with an alcohol pad and reuse.

BASICS   ASSESS   DISORDERS/   DRUGS/   DRUGS A-Z   CRISIS   GERI   TOOLS/

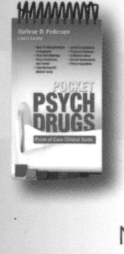
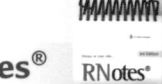
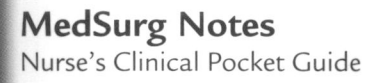
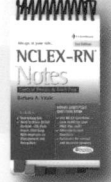
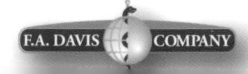

1

Mental Health and Mental Illness: Basics

Mental Health and Mental Illness: Basics

Mental health and mental illness have been defined in many ways but should always be viewed in the context of ethnocultural factors and influence.

Mental Illness/Disorder

The DSM-5 defines mental illness/disorder (paraphrased) as: *characterized by significant dysfunction in an individual's cognitions, emotions, or behaviors that reflects a disturbance in the psychological, biological, or developmental processes underlying mental functioning. A mental disorder is not merely an expectable or culturally sanctioned response to a specific event, such as the death of a loved one. The deviation from the norm is not political, religious, or sexual, but results from dysfunction in the individual (APA 2013).*

Mental Health

Mental health is defined as: *a state of successful performance of mental function, resulting in productive activities, fulfilling relationships with other people, and the ability to adapt to change and cope with adversity (US Surgeon General Report, Dec 1999).*

Wellness-illness continuum – Dunn's 1961 text, *High Level Wellness,* altered our concept of health and illness, viewing both as on a continuum that was dynamic and changing, focusing on levels of wellness. Concepts include: totality, uniqueness, energy, self-integration, energy use, and inner/outer worlds.

Legal Definition of Mental Illness

The legal definition of insanity/mental illness applies the M'Naghten Rule, formulated in 1843 and derived from English law. It says that: *a person is innocent by reason of insanity if at the time of committing the act, [the person] was laboring under a defect of reason from disease of the mind as not to know the nature and quality of the act being done, or if he did know it, he did not know that what he was doing was wrong.* There are variations of this legal definition by state, and some states have abolished the insanity defense.

Positive Mental Health: Jahoda's Six Major Categories

In 1958, Marie Jahoda developed six major categories of positive mental health:

- Attitudes of individual toward self
- Presence of growth and development, or actualization
- Personality integration

■ Autonomy and independence
■ Perception of reality, and
■ Environmental mastery

The mentally healthy person accepts the self, is self-reliant, and is self-confident.

Maslow's Hierarchy of Needs

Maslow developed a hierarchy of needs based on attainment of self-actualization, where one becomes highly evolved and attains his or her full potential.

The basic belief is that lower-level needs must be met first in order to advance to the next level of needs. Therefore, physiological and safety needs must be met before issues related to love and belonging can be addressed, through to self-actualization.

Maslow's Hierarchy of Needs	
Self-Actualization	Self-fulfillment/reach highest potential
Self-Esteem	Seek self-respect, achieve recognition
Love/Belonging	Giving/receiving affection, companionship
Safety and Security	Avoiding harm; order, structure, protection
Physiological	Air, water, food, shelter, sleep, elimination

General Adaptation Syndrome (Stress-Adaptation Syndrome)

Hans Selye (1976) divided his *stress syndrome* into three stages and, in doing so, pointed out the seriousness of prolonged stress on the body and the need for identification and intervention.

1. **Alarm stage** – This is the immediate physiological (fight or flight) response to a threat or perceived threat.
2. **Resistance** – If the stress continues, the body adapts to the levels of stress and attempts to return to homeostasis.
3. **Exhaustion** – With prolonged exposure and adaptation, the body eventually becomes depleted. There are no more reserves to draw upon, and serious illness may now develop (e.g., hypertension, mental disorders, cancer). Selye teaches us that without intervention, even death is a possibility at this stage.

CLINICAL PEARL: *Identification and treatment* of chronic, posttraumatic stress disorder (PTSD) and unresolved grief, including multiple (compounding) losses, are critical in an attempt to prevent serious illness and improve quality of life. (See PTSD table and PTSD Treatments in Disorders/Interventions tab and Military, Families, and PTSD in Crisis tab.)

Fight-or-Flight Response

In the fight-or-flight response, if a person is presented with a stressful situation (danger) a physiological response (sympathetic nervous system) activates the adrenal glands and cardiovascular system, allowing a person to adjust rapidly to the need to fight or flee in a situation.

- Such physiological response is beneficial in the short term; for instance, in an emergency situation.
- However, with ongoing, chronic psychological stressors, a person continues to experience the same physiological response as if there were a real danger, which eventually physically and emotionally depletes the body.

Diathesis-Stress Model

The diathesis-stress model views behavior as the result of *genetic* and *biological factors*. A genetic predisposition results in a mental disorder (e.g., mood disorder or schizophrenia) when precipitated by environmental factors.

Theories of Personality Development

Psychoanalytic Theory

Sigmund Freud, who introduced us to the Oedipus complex, hysteria, free association, and dream interpretation, is considered the "Father of Psychiatry." He was concerned with both the dynamics and structure of the psyche. He divided the personality into three parts:

- **Id** – The id developed out of Freud's concept of the pleasure principle.
  The id comprises primitive, instinctual drives (hunger, sex, aggression).
  The id says, "I want."
- **Ego** – It is the ego, or rational mind, that is called upon to control the instinctual impulses of the self-indulgent id. The ego says, "I think/I evaluate."
- **Superego** – The superego is the conscience of the psyche and monitors the ego. The superego says "I should/I ought" (Hunt 1994).

Topographic Model of the Mind

Freud's topographic model deals with levels of awareness and is divided into three categories:

- **Unconscious mind** – All mental content and memories *outside of conscious awareness;* becomes conscious through the preconscious mind.
- **Preconscious mind** – Not within the conscious mind but *can more easily be brought to conscious awareness* (repressive function of instinctual desires or undesirable memories). Reaches consciousness through word linkage.
- **Conscious mind** – All content and memories *immediately available and within conscious awareness.* Of lesser importance to psychoanalysts.

Key Defense Mechanisms

Defense Mechanism	Example
Denial – Refuses to accept a painful reality, pretending as if it doesn't exist.	A man who snorts cocaine daily is fired for attendance problems, yet insists he doesn't have a problem.
Displacement – Directing anger toward someone or onto another, less threatening (safer) substitute.	An older employee is publicly embarrassed by a younger boss at work and angrily cuts a driver off on the way home.
Identification – Taking on attributes and characteristics of someone admired.	A young man joins the police academy to become a policeman like his father, whom he respects.
Intellectualization – Excessive focus on logic and reason to avoid the feelings associated with a situation.	An executive who has cancer requests all studies and blood work and discusses in detail with her doctor, as if she were speaking about someone else.
Projection – Attributing to others feelings unacceptable to self.	A group therapy client strongly dislikes another member but claims that it is the member who "dislikes her."
Reaction Formation – Expressing an opposite feeling from what is actually felt and is considered undesirable.	John, who despises Jeremy, greets him warmly and offers him food and beverages and special attention.

Continued

Key Defense Mechanisms—cont'd

Defense Mechanism	Example
Sublimation – Redirecting unacceptable feelings or drives into an acceptable channel.	A mother of a child killed in a drive-by shooting becomes involved in legislative change for gun laws and gun violence.
Undoing – Ritualistically negating or undoing intolerable feelings/thoughts.	A man who has thoughts that his father will die must step on sidewalk cracks to prevent this and cannot miss a crack.

Stages of Personality Development

Freud's Psychosexual Development

Age	Stage	Task
0–18 mo	Oral	Oral gratification
18 mo–3 yr	Anal	Independence and control (voluntary sphincter control)
3–6 yr	Phallic	Genital focus
6–12 yr	Latency	Repressed sexuality; channeled sexual drives (sports)
13–20 yr	Genital	Puberty with sexual interest in opposite sex

Sullivan's Interpersonal Theory

Age	Stage	Task
0–18 mo	Infancy	Anxiety reduction via oral gratification
18 mo–6 yr	Childhood	Delay in gratification

Sullivan's Interpersonal Theory—cont'd

Age	Stage	Task
6–9 yr	Juvenile	Satisfying peer relationships
9–12 yr	Preadolescence	Satisfying same-sex relationships
12–14 yr	Early adolescence	Satisfying opposite-sex relationships
14–21 yr	Late adolescence	Lasting intimate opposite-sex relationship

Erikson's Psychosocial Theory

Age	Stage	Task
0–18 mo	Trust vs. mistrust	Basic trust in mother figure and generalizes
18 mo–3 yr	Autonomy vs. shame/doubt	Self-control/independence
3–6 yr	Initiative vs. guilt	Initiate and direct own activities
6–12 yr	Industry vs. inferiority	Self-confidence through successful performance and recognition
12–20 yr	Identity vs. role confusion	Task integration from previous stages; secure sense of self
20–30 yr	Intimacy vs. isolation	Form a lasting relationship or commitment
30–65 yr	Generativity vs. stagnation	Achieve life's goals; consider future generations
65 yr–death	Ego integrity vs. despair	Life review with meaning from both positives and negatives; positive self worth

Peplau's Interpersonal Theory

Age	Stage	Task
Infant	Depending on others	Learning ways to communicate with primary caregiver for meeting comfort needs
Toddler	Delaying satisfaction	Some delay in self-gratification to please others
Early Childhood	Self-identification	Acquisition of appropriate roles and behaviors through perception of others' expectations of self
Late Childhood	Participation skills	Competition, compromise, cooperation; skills acquisition; sense of one's place in the world

Stages of Personality Development tables modified from Townsend MC. Essentials of Psychiatric Mental Health Nursing, 6th ed. Philadelphia: FA Davis, 2014, used with permission

Mahler's Theory of Object Relations

Age	Phase (subphase)	Task
0–1 mo	1. Normal autism	Basic needs fulfillment (for survival)
1–5 mo	2. Symbiosis	Awareness of external fulfillment source
5–10 mo	3. Separation – individuation – Differentiation	Commencement of separateness from mother figure
10–16 mo	– Practicing	Locomotor independence; awareness of separateness of self
16–24 mo	– Rapprochement	Acute separateness awareness; seeks emotional refueling from mother figure
24–36 mo	– Consolidation	Established sense of separateness; internalizes sustained image of loved person/object when out of sight; separation anxiety resolution

Biological Aspects of Mental Illness

Mind-Body Dualism to Brain and Behavior

- René Descartes (17th C) espoused the theory of the mind-body dualism (Cartesian dualism), wherein the mind (soul) was said to be completely separate from the body.
- Current research and approaches show the connection between mind and body and that newer treatments will develop from a better understanding of both the biological and psychological (Hunt 1994).
- The US Congress stated that the 1990s would be "The Decade of the Brain," with increased focus and research in the areas of neurobiology, genetics, and biological markers.
- The Decade of Behavior (2000–2010) is a "multidisciplinary" initiative launched by the American Psychological Association (APA), focusing on the behavioral and social sciences, trying to address major challenges facing the US today in health, safety, education, prosperity, and democracy (www.decadeofbehavior.org).

Central and Peripheral Nervous System

Central Nervous System

- Brain
  - Forebrain:
    - *Cerebrum (frontal, parietal, temporal, and occipital lobes)*
    - *Diencephalon (thalamus, hypothalamus, and limbic system)*
  - Midbrain
    - *Mesencephalon*
  - Hindbrain
    - Pons, medulla, and cerebellum
- Nerve Tissue
  - Neurons
  - Synapses
  - Neurotransmitters
- Spinal Cord
  - Fiber tracts
  - Spinal nerves

Continued

Peripheral Nervous System

■ Afferent System
   ■ Sensory neurons (somatic and visceral)
■ Efferent System
   ■ Somatic nervous system (somatic motor neurons)
   ■ Autonomic nervous system
   ■ Sympathetic nervous system
      Visceral motor neurons
   • Parasympathetic nervous system
      Visceral motor neurons

The Brain

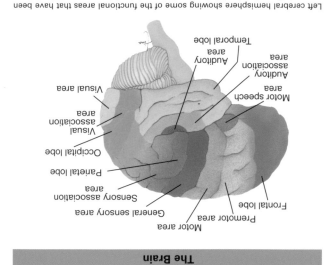

Left cerebral hemisphere showing some of the functional areas that have been mapped. (From Scanlon VC, Sanders T. Essentials of Anatomy and Physiology, 6th ed. Philadelphia: FA Davis; 2011, used with permission)

Limbic System

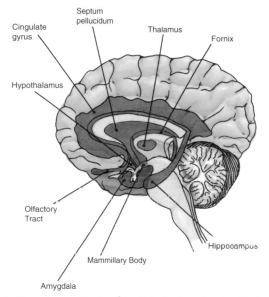

The limbic system and its structures. (Adapted from Scanlon VC, Sanders T. Essentials of Anatomy and Physiology, 6th ed. FA Davis: Philadelphia, 2011, used with permission)

Autonomic Nervous System

Sympathetic and Parasympathetic Effects

Structure	Sympathetic	Parasympathetic
Eye (pupil)	Dilation	Constriction
Nasal Mucosa	Mucus reduction	Mucus increased
Salivary Gland	Saliva reduction	Saliva increased
Heart	Rate increased	Rate decreased
Arteries	Constriction	Dilation
Lung	Bronchial muscle relaxation	Bronchial muscle contraction
Gastrointestinal Tract	Decreased motility	Increased motility
Liver	Conversion of glycogen to glucose increased	Glycogen synthesis
Kidney	Decreased urine	Increased urine
Bladder	Contraction of sphincter	Relaxation of sphincter
Sweat Glands	↓ Sweating	No change

Synapse Transmission

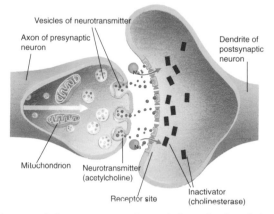

Impulse transmission at a synapse. Arrows indicate direction of electrical impulse. (From Scanlon VC, Sanders T. Essentials of Anatomy and Physiology, 6th ed. FA Davis: Philadelphia, 2011, used with permission)

Neurotransmitters

Neurotransmitter Functions and Effects

Neurotransmitter	Function	Effect
Dopamine	Inhibitory	Fine movement, emotional behavior. Implicated in schizophrenia and Parkinson's.
Serotonin	Inhibitory	Sleep, mood, eating behavior. Implicated in mood disorders, anxiety, and violence.

Continued

Neurotransmitter Functions and Effects—cont'd

Neurotransmitter	Function	Effect
Norepinephrine	Excitatory	Arousal, wakefulness, learning. Implicated in anxiety and addiction.
Gamma-aminobutyric acid (GABA)	Inhibitory	Anxiety states.
Acetylcholine	Excitatory	Arousal, attention, movement. Increase = spasms and decrease = paralysis.

Legal-Ethical Issues

Confidentiality

Confidentiality in all of health care is important but notably so in psychiatry because of possible discriminatory treatment of those with mental illness. All individuals have a right to privacy, and all client records and communications should be kept confidential.

Do's and Don'ts of Confidentiality

■ Do not discuss clients by using their actual names or any identifier that could be linked to a particular client (e.g., name/date of birth on an x-ray/ assessment form).

■ Do not discuss client particulars outside of a private, professional environment. Do not discuss with family members or friends.

■ Be particularly careful in elevators of hospitals or community centers. You never know who might be on the elevator with you.

■ Even in educational presentations, protect client identity by changing names (John Doe) and obtaining all (informed consent) permissions.

■ Every client has the right to confidential and respectful treatment.

■ Accurate, objective record keeping is important, and documentation is significant in demonstrating what was actually done for client care. If not documented, treatments are not considered done.

When Confidentiality Must Be Breached

Confidentiality and Child Abuse – If it is suspected or clear that a child is being abused or in danger of abuse (physical/sexual/emotional) or neglect, the health professional must report such abuse as mandated by the Child Abuse Prevention Treatment Act, originally enacted in 1974 (PL 93-247).

Confidentiality and Elder Abuse – If suspected or clear that an elder is being abused or in danger of abuse or neglect, then the health professional must also report this abuse.

■ ***Tarasoff Principle/Duty to Warn*** (*Tarasoff v. Regents* of the University of California 1976) – Refers to the responsibility of a therapist, health professional, or nurse to warn a potential victim of imminent danger (a threat to harm person) and breach confidentiality. **The person in danger and others (able to protect person) must be notified of the intended harm.**

The Health Insurance Portability and Accountability Act (HIPAA) (1996)

Enacted on August 21, 1996, HIPAA was established with the goal of assuring that an individual's health information is properly protected while allowing the flow of health information (US Department of Health and Human Services 2006; HIPAA 2006).

Types of Commitment

■ **Voluntary** – An individual decides treatment is needed and admits himself/herself to a hospital, leaving of own volition – unless a professional (psychiatrist/other professional) decides that the person is a danger to himself/herself or others.

■ **Involuntary** – Involuntary commitments include: 1) emergency commitments, including those unable to care for self (basic personal needs), and 2) involuntary outpatient commitment (IOC).

■ ***Emergency*** – Involves ***imminent*** danger to self or others; has demonstrated a ***clear and present danger to self or others.*** Usually initiated by health professionals, authorities, and sometimes friends or family. Person is threatening to harm self or others. Or evidence that the person is unable to care for herself or himself (nourishment, personal, medical, safety) with reasonable probability that death will result within a month.

■ ***302 Emergency Involuntary Commitment*** – If a person is an *immediate danger to self or others* or is *in danger due to a lack of ability to care for self*, then an emergency psychiatric evaluation may be filed (section 302). This person must then be evaluated by a psychiatrist and released, or psychiatrist may uphold petition (patient admitted for up to 5 days) (Emergency commitments 2004; Christy et al 2010).

Restraints and Seclusion for an Adult — Behavioral Health Care

The Joint Commission on Accreditation of Healthcare Organizations (JCAHO) wants to reduce the use of behavioral restraints but has set forth guidelines for safety in the event they are used.

■ In an emergency situation, restraints may be applied by an authorized and qualified staff member, but an order must be obtained from a Licensed Independent Practitioner (LIP) within 1 hour of initiation of restraints/seclusion.

■ Following application of restraints, the following time frames must be adhered to for reevaluation/reordering:

...wa in st nod, physician et al. must evaluate the patient face-to-face after initiation of restraint/seclusion, if hospital uses accreditation for Medicare-deemed status purposes. If not for deemed status, LIP performs face-to-face evaluation within 4 hours of initiation of restraint/seclusion.

- If adult is released prior to expiration of original order, LIP must perform a face-to-face evaluation within 24 hours of initiation of restraint/seclusion.
- LIP reorders restraint every 4 hours until adult is released from restraint/seclusion. A qualified RN or other authorized staff person reevaluates individual status and need to continue restraint/seclusion.
- LIP face-to-face evaluation every 8 hours until patient is released from restraint/seclusion.
- 4-hour RN or other qualified staff reassessment and 8-hour face-to-face evaluation repeated, as long as restraint/seclusion clinically necessary (JCAHO revised 2009).
- The *American Psychiatric Nurses Association* and *International Society of Psychiatric-Mental Health Nurses* are committed to the *reduction of seclusion and restraint* and have developed position statements, with a vision of eventually eliminating seclusion and restraint (APNA 2007; ISPN 1999).

Learn your institutional policies on restraints and seclusion and take advantage of any training available, contacting supervisors/managers if any questions about protocols.

🚫 **ALERT:** The decision to initiate seclusion or restraint is made only after all other less restrictive, nonphysical methods have failed to resolve the behavioral emergency (APNA 2001). Restraint of a patient may be both physical and pharmacological (chemical) and infringes on a patient's freedom of movement and may result in injury (physical or psychological) and/or death. There must be an evaluation based on benefit: risk consideration and a leaning toward alternative solutions. Restraints may be used when there is dangerous behavior and to protect the patient and others. You need to become familiar with the standards as set forth by JCAHO and any state regulations and hospital policies. *The least restrictive method should be used and considered first, before using more restrictive interventions.*

A Patient's Bill of Rights
- First adopted in 1973 by the American Hospital Association, A Patient's Bill of Rights was revised on October 21, 1992.
- Sets forth an expectation of treatment and care that will allow for improved collaboration between patients, health care providers, and institutions resulting in better patient care (American Hospital Association [revised] 1992).

The Patient Care Partnership
In 2003 "A Patient's Bill of Rights" was replaced by "The Patient Care Partnership," in order to emphasize the collaboration between patient and health providers (American Hospital Association 2003).

Quality and Safety Education for Nurses (QSEN)

The Quality and Safety Education for Nurses (QSEN) project (2005), funded by the Robert Wood Johnson Foundation, focused on the promotion of quality and safety in patient care. Teaching strategies include the following core competencies, which are needed to develop student and graduate attitudes and skills for quality patient care and safety: evidence-based practice, safety, teamwork and collaboration, patient-centered care, quality improvement and informatics (QSEN 2012). Additional information, including QSEN teaching strategies, can be found in Townsend: Essentials of Psychiatric Mental Health Nursing, 6th ed., 2014 and other resources.

Informed Consent

- Every adult person has the right to decide what can and cannot be done to his or her own body (*Schloendorff v. Society of New York Hospital*, 105 NE 92 [NY 1914]).
- Assumes a person is capable of making an informed decision about own health care.
- State regulations vary, but mental illness does not mean that a person is or should be assumed incapable of making decisions related to his or her own care.
- Patients have a right to:
  - Information about their treatment and any procedures to be performed.
  - Know the inherent risks and benefits.

Without this information (specific information, risks, and benefits) a person cannot make an informed decision. The above also holds true for those who might participate in research. Videocasts on informed consent can be accessed at: http://videocast.nih.gov (National Institutes of Health, Informed Consent: The ideal and the reality, Session 5 November 9, 2005).

Right to Refuse Treatment/Medication

- Just as a person has the right to accept treatment, he or she also has the right to refuse treatment to the extent permitted by the law and to be informed of the medical consequences of his/her actions.
- In some emergency situations, a patient can be medicated or treated against his/her will, but state laws vary, and so it is imperative to become knowledgeable about applicable state laws (American Hospital Association [revised] 1992; American Hospital Association 2003).

Health Care Reform and Behavioral Health

On March 23, 2010, President Barack Obama signed into law a comprehensive health care and reform legislation. Extensive information can be found at: http://mentalhealthcarereform.org. This site explains and summarizes the law, provides timelines for implementation, discusses health reform and parity, and provides excellent links to other relevant organizations. The American Psychiatric Association has approved a position statement entitled Principles for Health Care Reform for Psychiatry (2008). It is important to keep current as to mental health care reform, par-

Psychiatric Assessment

Psychiatric History and Assessment Tool

Identifying/Demographic Information

Name _____ Room No. _____

Primary Care Provider: _____

DOB _____ Age_____ Sex _____

Race: _____ Ethnicity: _____

Marital Status: _____ No. Marriages: _____

If married/divorced/separated/widowed, how long? _____

Occupation/School (grade): _____ _____

Highest Education Level: _____

Religious Affiliation: _____

City of Residence: _____

Name/Phone # of Significant Other: _____

Primary Language Spoken: _____ _____

Accompanied by: _____ _____

Admitted from: _____ _____

Previous Psychiatric Hospitalizations (#): _____

Chief Complaint (in patient's own words): _____

DSM-5 Diagnosis (previous/current): ___ _____

Nursing Diagnosis: _____

Notes:

Family Members/Significant Others Living in Home

Name	Relationship	Age	Occupation/Grade

Family Members/Significant Others Not in Home

Name	Relationship	Age	Occupation/Grade

Children

Name	Age	Living at Home?

CLINICAL PEARL: Compare what the client says with what other family members, friends, or significant others say about situations or previous treatments. It is usually helpful to gather information from those who have observed/lived with the client and can provide *another valuable source/side of information*. The *reliability of the client* in recounting the past must be considered and should be noted.

Genogram—See *Disorders/Intervention Tab* for sample genogram and common genogram symbols.

Past Psychiatric Treatments/Medications

It is important to obtain a history of any previous psychiatric hospitalizations, the number of hospitalizations and dates, and to record all current/past psychotropic medications, as well as other medications the client may be taking. Ask the client what has worked in the past, and also what has *not* worked, for both treatments and medications.

Inpatient Treatment

Facility/Location	Dates From/To	Diagnosis	Treatments	Response(s)

Outpatient Treatments/Services

Psychiatrist/Therapist	Location	Diagnosis	Treatment	Response(s)

Psychotropic Medications (Previous Treatments)

Name	Dose/Dosages	Treatment Length	Response	Comments

Current Psychotropic Medications

Name	Dose/Dosages	Date Started	Response(s)	Serum Levels

Other Current Medications, Herbals, and OTC Medications

Name	Dose/ Dosages	Date Started	Response(s)	Comments

CLINICAL PEARL: It is important to ask about any herbals, OTC medications (e.g., pseudoephedrine), or nontraditional treatments as client may not think to mention these when questioned about current medications. *Important herbals include, but are not limited to:* St. John's wort, ephedra (ma huang), ginseng, kava kava, and yohimbe. These can interact with psychotropics or other medications or cause anxiety and/or drowsiness, as well as other adverse physiological reactions. Be sure to record and then report any additional or herbal medications to the psychiatrist, advanced practice nurse, psychiatric nurse, and professional team staff.

Medical History (*See Clinical Pearls for Italics*)

TPR:		BP:	
Height:		Weight:	

Cardiovascular (CV)

Does client have or ever had the following disorders/symptoms (include date):

Hypertension	Murmurs	Chest Pain (Angina)
Palpitations/ Tachycardia	Shortness of Breath	Ankle Edema/Congestive Heart Failure
Fainting/Syncope	Myocardial Infarction	High Cholesterol
Leg Pain (Claudication)	*Arrhythmias*	*Other CV Disease*
Heart Bypass	Angioplasty	Other CV surgery

CLINICAL PEARL: Heterocyclic antidepressants must be used with caution with *cardiovascular disease*. Tricyclic antidepressants (TCAs) may produce life-threatening *arrhythmias* and ECG changes.

Central Nervous System (CNS)

Does client have or ever had the following disorders/symptoms (include date):

Headache	Head Injury	Tremors
Dizziness/Vertigo	Loss of Consciousness (LOC); how long?	Stroke
Myasthenia Gravis	Parkinson's Disease	Dementia
Brain Tumor	Seizure Disorder	Multiple Sclerosis
TIAs	Other	Surgery

CLINICAL PEARL: Remember that *myasthenia gravis* is a contraindication to the use of antipsychotics; *tremors* could be due to a disease such as *Parkinson's* or could be a side effect of a psychotropic (lithium/antipsychotic). Sometimes the elderly may be diagnosed as having *dementia* when in fact they are depressed (pseudodementia). Use TCAs cautiously with *seizure disorders;* bupropion use contraindicated in seizure disorder.

Dermatological/Skin

Does client have or ever had the following disorders/symptoms (include date):

Psoriasis	Hair Loss	Itching
Rashes	Acne	Other/Surgeries

CLINICAL PEARL: Lithium can precipitate psoriasis or psoriatic arthritis in patients with a history of *psoriasis*, or the psoriasis may be new onset. *Acne* is also a possible reaction to lithium (new onset or exacerbation), and lithium may result in, although rarely, *hair loss (alopecia)*. *Rashes* in patients on carbamazepine or lamotrigine may be a sign of a life-threatening mucocutaneous reaction, such as Stevens-Johnson syndrome (SJS). Discontinue medication/immediate medical attention needed.

Endocrinology/Metabolic

Does client have or ever had the following disorders/symptoms (include date):

Polydipsia	Polyuria	Diabetes Type 1 or 2
Hyperthyroidism	*Hypothyroidism*	Hirsutism
Polycystic Ovarian Syndrome	Other	Surgery

CLINICAL PEARL: Clients on lithium should be observed and tested for hypothyroidism. Atypical and older antipsychotics are associated with treatment-emergent diabetes (need periodic testing; FBS, HgbA1c, lipids; BMI, etc).

Eye, Ears, Nose, Throat

Does client have or ever had the following disorders/symptoms (include date):

Eye Pain	*Halo around Light Source*	*Blurring*
Red Eye	Double vision	Flashing Lights/ Floaters
Glaucoma	Tinnitus	Ear Pain/Otitis Media
Hoarseness	Other	Other/Surgery

CLINICAL PEARL: *Eye pain and halo around a light source are possible symptoms of glaucoma. Closed-angle glaucoma* is a true emergency and requires immediate medical attention to prevent blindness. Anticholinergics (low-potency antipsychotics [chlorpromazine] or tricyclics) can cause *blurred vision.* Check for history of *glaucoma* as antipsychotics are contraindicated.

Gastrointestinal

Does client have or ever had the following disorders/symptoms (include date):

Nausea & Vomiting	Diarrhea	Constipation
GERD	Crohn's Disease	Colitis
Colon Cancer	Irritable Bowel Syndrome	Other/Surgery

CLINICAL PEARL: *Nausea* is a common side effect of many medications; tricyclic antidepressants can cause *constipation*. Nausea seems to be more common with paroxetine. Over time clients may adjust to these side effects, therefore no decision should be made about effectiveness/side effects or changing medications without a reasonable trial.

Genitourinary/Reproductive

Does client have or ever had the following disorders/symptoms (include date):

Miscarriages? Y/N		Abortions? Y/N	
# When?		# When?	
Nipple Discharge	Amenorrhea	Gynecomastia	
Lactation	Dysuria	Urinary Incontinence	
Pregnancy Problems	Postpartum Depression	Sexual Dysfunction	
Prostate Problems (BPH)	Menopause	Fibrocystic Breast Disease	
Penile Discharge	UTI	Pelvic Pain	
Renal Disease	Urinary Cancer	Breast Cancer	
Other/Surgery Cancer	Other Gynecological	Other	

CLINICAL PEARL: Antipsychotics have an effect on the endocrinological system by affecting the tuberoinfundibular system. Those on antipsychotics may experience *gynecomastia and lactation (men also)*. Women may experience *amenorrhea*. Some drugs (TCAs), such as amitriptyline, must be used with caution with BPH. *Postpartum depression* requires evaluation and treatment (*see Postpartum Major Depressive Episode in Disorders-Interventions Tab*). **Men should also be observed/evaluated for postpartum depression.**

Respiratory

Does client have or ever had (include date):

Chronic Cough	Sore Throat	Bronchitis
Asthma	COPD	Pneumonia
Cancer (Lung/Throat)	Sleep Apnea	Other/Surgery

Other Questions:

Allergies (food/environmental/pet/contact)

_____

Diet _____

Drug Allergies _____

Accidents _____

High Prolonged Fever _____

Tobacco Use _____

Childhood Illnesses _____

Fractures _____

Menses Began _____

Birth Control _____

Disabilities (hearing/speech/movement) _____

Pain (describe/location/length of time [over or under 3 months]/severity between 1 [least] and 10 [worst])/Treatment

_____

Family History

Mental Illness _____

_____

Medical Disorders _____

_____

Substance Abuse _____

Please note who in the family has the problem/disorder.

Substance Use
Prescribed Drugs

Name	Dosage	Reason

Street Drugs

Name	Amount/Day	Reason

Alcohol

Name	Amount/Day/Week	Reason

Substance History and Assessment Tool

1. When you were growing up, did anyone in your family use substances (alcohol or drugs)? If yes, how did the substance use affect the family?

2. When (how old) did you use your first substance (e.g., alcohol, cannabis) and what was it?

3. How long have you been using a substance(s) regularly? Weeks, months, years?

4. Pattern of abuse
   a. When do you use substances?
   b. How much and how often do you use?
   c. Where are you when you use substances and with whom?

5. When did you last use; what was it and how much did you use?

6. Has substance use caused you any problems with family, friends, job, school, the legal system, other? If yes, describe:

7. Have you ever had an injury or accident because of substance abuse? If yes, describe:

8. Have you ever been arrested for a DUI because of your drinking or other substance use?

9. Have you ever been arrested or placed in jail because of drugs or alcohol?

10. Have you ever experienced memory loss the morning after substance use (can't remember what you did the night before? Describe the event and feelings about the situation:

11. Have you ever tried to stop your substance use? If yes, why were you not able to stop? Did you have any physical symptoms such as shakiness, sweating, nausea, headaches, insomnia, or seizures?

12. Describe a typical day in your life.

13. Are there any changes you would like to make in your life? If so, describe:

14. What plans or ideas do you have for making these changes?

15. History of withdrawal:
    Other comments:

Modified from Townsend 6th ed., 2014, with permission

Short Michigan Alcohol Screening Test (SMAST)

- Do you feel you are a normal drinker? [no] Y__ N__
- Does someone close to you worry about your drinking? [yes] Y__ N__
- Do you feel guilty about your drinking? [yes] Y__ N__
- Do friends/relatives think you're a normal drinker? [no] Y__ N__
- Can you stop drinking when you want to? [no] Y__ N__
- Have you ever attended an AA meeting? [yes] Y__ N__
- Has drinking created problems between you and a loved one/relative? [yes] Y__ N__
- Gotten in trouble at work because of drinking? [yes] Y__ N__
- Neglected obligations/family/work 2 days in a row because of drinking? [yes] Y__ N__
- Gone to anyone for help for your drinking? [yes] Y__ N__
- Ever been in a hospital because of drinking? [yes] Y__ N__
- Arrested for drunk driving or DUI? [yes] Y__ N__
- Arrested for other drunken behavior? [yes] Y__ N__
- Total =

Five or more positive items suggest alcohol problem.
(Positive answers are in brackets above) (Selzer 1975)

Mental Status Assessment and Tool

The components of the mental status assessment are:

- General Appearance
- Behavior/Activity
- Speech and Language
- Mood and Affect
- Thought Process and Content
- Perceptual Disturbances
- Memory/Cognitive
- Judgment and Insight

Each component must be approached in a methodical manner so that a thorough evaluation of the client can be done from a mood, thought, appearance, insight, judgment, and overall perspective. It is important to document all these findings even though this record represents one point in time. It is helpful over time to see any patterns (regressions/improvement) and to gain an understanding of any changes that would trigger a need to reevaluate the client or suggest a decline in functioning.

Mental Status Assessment Tool

Identifying Information

Name	Age
Sex	Race/Ethnicity
Significant Other	Educational Level
Religion	Occupation

Presenting problem:

Appearance

Grooming/dress _____

Hygiene _____

Eye contact _____

Continued

Mental Status Assessment Tool—cont'd

Posture _____

Identifying features (marks/scars/tattoos) _____

Appearance versus stated age _____

Overall appearance _____

CLINICAL PEARL: It is helpful to ask the client to talk about him/herself and to *ask open-ended questions* to help the client express thoughts and feelings; e.g., "Tell me why you are here?" Encourage further discussion with: "Tell me more." A less direct and more conversational tone at the beginning of the interview may help reduce the client's anxiety and set the stage for the trust needed in a therapeutic relationship.

Behavior/Activity (check if present)

Hyperactive _____

Agitated _____

Psychomotor retardation _____

Calm _____

Tremors_____

Tics _____

Unusual movements/gestures _____

Catatonia _____

Akathisia _____

Rigidity _____

Facial movements (jaw/lip smacking) _____

Other _____

Speech

Slow/rapid _____

Pressured _____

Tone_____

Volume (loud/soft) _____

Fluency (mute/hesitation/latency of response) _____

Continued

Attitude

Is client:

Cooperative _____	Uncooperative _____
Warm/friendly _____	Distant _____
Suspicious _____	Combative _____
Guarded _____	Aggressive _____
Hostile _____	Aloof _____
Apathetic _____	Other _____

Mood and Affect

Is client:

Elated _____	Sad _____	Depressed _____
Anxious _____	Irritable _____	
Fearful _____	Guilty _____	
Worried _____	Angry _____	
Hopeless _____	Labile _____	

Mixed (anxious and depressed) _____

Is client's affect:

Flat _____

Blunted or diminished _____

Appropriate _____

Inappropriate/incongruent (sad and smiling/laughing) _____

Other _____

Thought Process

Concrete thinking _____

Circumstantiality _____

Tangentiality _____

Loose association _____

Echolalia _____

Flight of ideas _____

Perseveration _____

Clang associations _____

Blocking _____

Word salad _____

Derailment _____

Other _____

Thought Content

Does client have:

Delusions (grandiose/persecution/reference/somatic): _____

_____

Suicidal/homicidal thoughts _____

If homicidal, toward whom? (Must report and notify intended victim)

_____

Obsessions_____

Paranoia _____

Phobias _____

Magical thinking _____

Poverty of speech _____

Other _____

CLINICAL PEARL: Questions around suicide and homicide need to be direct. For instance, *Are you thinking of harming yourself/another person right now?* (If another, who?) Clients will usually admit to suicidal thoughts *if asked directly* but will not always volunteer this information. Any threat to harm someone else requires informing the potential victim and the authorities. *(See When Confidentiality Must Be Breached, Tarasoff Principle/Duty to Warn, in Basics Tab.)*

Perceptual Disturbances

Is client experiencing:

Visual Hallucinations _____

Auditory Hallucinations _____

    Commenting _____

    Discussing _____

    Commanding

    Loud _____

    Soft _____

    Other _____

Other Hallucination (olfactory/tactile) _____

Continued

| Illusions _____ |
| Depersonalization _____ |
| Other _____ |

Memory/Cognitive
Orientation (time/place/person)_____

Memory (recent/remote/confabulation) _____

Level of alertness _____

Insight and Judgment
Insight (awareness of the nature of the illness)_____

Judgment _____

For example: "What would you do if you saw a fire in a movie theater?"

Other _____

Impulse control _____

Other _____

Multiaxial Assessment

The DSM-5 (APA 2013) will no longer use the 5-axis multiaxial assessment tool, now combining axes I (clinical diagnosis), II (personality disorder/intellectual disability), and III (general medical conditions) for listing a diagnosis. Former axes IV (psychosocial factors) and V (GAF/functional disability) will be replaced with notations (using ICD-9/10-CM V and Z codes) about those factors.

Abnormal Involuntary Movement Scale (AIMS)

- ■ AIMS is a 5- to 10-minute clinician/other-trained rater (psychiatric nurse) scale to assess for tardive dyskinesia. AIMS is not a scored scale but rather a comparative scale documenting changes over time (Guy 1976).
- ■ Baseline should be done before instituting pharmacotherapy and then every 3 to 6 months thereafter. Check with federal and hospital regulations for time frames. Long-term care facilities are required to perform the AIMS at initiation of antipsychotic therapy and every 6 months thereafter.

AIMS Examination Procedure
Either before or after completing the examination procedure, observe the client unobtrusively, at rest (e.g., in waiting room). The chair to be used in this examination should be hard and firm without arms.

- Ask client to remove shoes and socks.
- Ask client if there is anything in his/her mouth (e.g., gum, candy); if there is, to remove it.
- Ask client about the current condition of his/her teeth. Ask client if he/she wears dentures. Do teeth or dentures bother the client now?
- Ask client whether he/she notices any movements in mouth, face, hands, or feet. If yes, ask to describe and to what extent they currently bother client or interfere with his/her activities.
- Have client sit in chair with hands on knees, legs slightly apart and feet flat on floor. (Look at entire body for movements while client is in this position.)
- Ask client to sit with hands hanging unsupported: if male, between legs; if female and wearing a dress, hanging over knees. (Observe hands and other body areas.)
- Ask client to open mouth. (Observe tongue at rest in mouth.) Do this twice.
- Ask client to protrude tongue. (Observe abnormalities of tongue movement.) Do this twice.
- Ask client to tap thumb, with each finger, as rapidly as possible for 10 to 15 seconds; separately with right hand, then with left hand. (Observe facial and leg movements.)
- Flex and extend client's left and right arms (one at a time). (Note any rigidity.)
- Ask client to stand up. (Observe in profile. Observe all body areas again, hips included.)
- Ask client to extend both arms outstretched in front with palms down. (Observe trunk, legs, and mouth.)
- Have client walk a few paces, turn, and walk back to chair. (Observe hands and gait.) Do this twice.

AIMS Rating Form	
Name	Rater Name
Date	ID #
Instructions: Complete the above examination procedure before making ratings. For movement ratings, circle the highest severity observed.	Code. 0: None 1: Minimal, may be extreme normal 2: Mild 3: Moderate 4: Severe

Continued

AIMS Rating Form—cont'd

Facial and Oral Movements	**1. Muscles of Facial Expression** • e.g., movements of forehead, eyebrows, periorbital area, cheeks • include frowning, blinking, smiling, and grimacing	0 1 2 3 4
	2. Lips and Perioral Area • e.g., puckering, pouting, smacking	0 1 2 3 4
	3. Jaw • e.g., biting, clenching, chewing, mouth opening, lateral movement	0 1 2 3 4
	4. Tongue • Rate only increase in movements both in and out of the mouth, NOT the inability to sustain movement	0 1 2 3 4
Extremity Movements	**5. Upper** *(arms, wrists, hands, fingers)* • Include choreic movements (i.e., rapid, objectively purposeless, irregular, spontaneous), athetoid movements (i.e., slow, irregular, complex, serpentine). • Do NOT include tremor (i.e., repetitive, regular, rhythmic).	0 1 2 3 4
Trunk Movements	**6. Lower** *(legs, knees, ankles, toes)* • e.g., lateral knee movement, foot tapping, heel dropping, foot squirming, inversion and eversion of the foot	0 1 2 3 4
	7. Neck, shoulders, hips • e.g., rocking, twisting, squirming, pelvic gyrations	0 1 2 3 4
Global Judgments	**8. Severity of Abnormal Movements**	0 1 2 3 4
	9. Incapacitation Due to Abnormal Movements	0 1 2 3 4
	10. Client's Awareness of Abnormal Movements • Rate only client's report.	0 1 2 3 4

AIMS Rating Form—cont'd

| **Dental Status** | 11. **Current Problems With Teeth and/or Dentures** | 0: No 1: Yes |
| | 12. **Does Client Usually Wear Dentures?** | 0: No 1: Yes |

The Edinburgh Postnatal Depression Scale (EPDS)

The EPDS is a valid screening tool for detecting postpartum depression. It is important to differentiate postpartum blues from postpartal depression and to observe for psychosis. Bipolar disorder and previous postpartum psychosis increase risk for suicide or infanticide. (See *Postpartum Major Depressive Episode* in the Disorders-Interventions Tab for signs and symptoms, evaluation, and treatment of postpartum depression.) **Note:** May also be used to screen for paternal depression (Edmondson 2010).

The Edinburgh Postnatal Depression Scale (EPDS)

Name: _____

Your date of birth: _____

Baby's Age: _____

As you have recently had a baby, we would like to know how you are feeling now. Please underline the answer that comes closest to how you have felt IN THE PAST 7 DAYS, not just how you feel today.

Sample question:
Here is an example already completed:
I have felt happy
• Yes, most of the time
• Yes, some of the time
• No, not very often
• No, not at all

This would mean "I have felt happy some of the time during the past week."
Please complete the following questions in the same way:

1. I have been able to laugh and see the funny side of things.
   • As much as I always could
   • Not quite so much now
   • Definitely not so much now
   • Not at all

2. I have looked forward with enjoyment to things.
   • As much as I ever did
   • Rather less than I used to
   • Definitely less than I used to
   • Hardly at all

The Edinburgh Postnatal Depression Scale (EPDS)—cont'd

3. I have blamed myself unnecessarily when things went wrong.*
   • Yes, most of the time
   • Yes, some of the time
   • Not very often
   • No, never

4. I have been anxious or worried for no good reason.
   • No, not at all
   • Hardly ever
   • Yes, sometimes
   • Yes, very often

5. I have felt scared or panicky for no very good reason.*
   • Yes, quite a lot
   • Yes, sometimes
   • No, not much
   • No, not at all

6. Things have been getting on top of me.*
   • Yes, most of the time I haven't been able to cope at all
   • Yes, sometimes I haven't been coping as well as usual
   • No, most of the time I have coped quite well
   • No, I have been coping as well as ever

7. I have been so unhappy that I have had difficulty sleeping.*
   • Yes, most of the time
   • Yes, sometimes
   • Not very often
   • No, not at all

8. I have felt sad or miserable.*
   • Yes, most of the time
   • Yes, quite often
   • Not very often
   • No, not at all

9. I have been so unhappy that I have been crying.*
   • Yes, most of the time
   • Yes, quite often
   • Only occasionally
   • No, never

10. The thought of harming myself has occurred to me.*
   • Yes, quite often
   • Sometimes
   • Hardly ever
   • Never

Total score = _____ (See scoring on following page)

Instructions for users:

1. The mother is asked to underline the response that comes closest to how she has been feeling in the previous 7 days.
2. All ten items must be completed.
3. Care should be taken to avoid the possibility of the mother discussing her answers with others.
4. The mother should complete the scale herself, unless she has limited English or has difficulty with reading.
5. The EPDS may be used at 6–8 weeks to screen postnatal women. The child health clinic, postnatal check-up, or a home visit may provide suitable opportunities for its completion.

Scoring:

Questions 1, 2, and 4 are scored 0, 1, 2, and 3 according to increased severity of the symptoms. The top response (e.g., As much as I always could, question 1) would be scored a 0 and the bottom response (e.g., Not at all, question 1) scored a 3. Items marked with an asterisk * (questions 3, 5–10) are reverse scored (i.e., 3, 2, 1, and 0). The total score is calculated by adding together the scores for each of the ten items. Maximum score is 30. Patients scoring 13 or more should be assessed for possible depression. A cut-off of 10 or more may be used if greater sensitivity is required. Any score above 0 on item 10 should always prompt further assessment.

SOURCE: © 1987 The Royal College of Psychiatrists. The Edinburgh Post-natal Depression Scale may be photocopied by individual researchers or clinicians for their own use without seeking permission from the publishers. The scale must be copied in full and all copies must acknowledge the following source: Cox JL, Holden JM, Sagovsky R. Detection of postnatal depression. Development of the 10-item Edinburgh Postnatal Depression Scale. British Journal of Psychiatry 1987; 150:782–786. Written permission must be obtained from the Royal College of Psychiatrists for copying and distribution to others or for republication (in print, online or by any other medium).

Translations of the scale, and guidance as to its use, may be found in Cox JL, Holden J. Perinatal Mental Health: A Guide to the Edinburgh Postnatal Depression Scale. London: Gaskell, 2003.

Scoring for Men:

A score of greater than 10 was found to be the optimal cutoff for men and shown to have a reasonable sensitivity and specificity (Edmondson 2010).

Hamilton Depression Rating Scale (HAM-D)

A clinician rated scale to rate the severity of depression.
For each item, circle the number to select the one "cue" that best characterizes the patient.

1. **Depressed Mood** (sadness, hopeless, helpless, worthless)
   0 = Absent.
   1 = These feeling states indicated only on questioning.
   2 = These feeling states spontaneously reported verbally.
   3 = Communicates feeling states nonverbally, i.e., through facial expression, posture, voice, tendency to weep.
   4 = Patient reports virtually only these feeling states in spontaneous verbal and nonverbal communication.

2. **Feelings of Guilt**
   0 = Absent.
   1 = Self reproach; feels he/she has let people down.
   2 = Ideas of guilt or rumination over past errors or sinful deeds.
   3 = Present illness is a punishment. Delusions of guilt.
   4 = Hears accusatory or denunciatory voices and/or experiences threatening visual hallucinations.

Continued

3. **Suicide**
   0 = Absent.
   1 = Feels life is not worth living.
   2 = Wishes he/she were dead or any thoughts of possible death to self.
   3 = Suicidal ideas or gesture.
   4 = Attempts at suicide (any serious attempt rates 4).

4. **Insomnia: Early in the Night**
   0 = No difficulty falling asleep.
   1 = Complains of occasional difficulty falling asleep, i.e., more than $1/2$ hour.
   2 = Complains of nightly difficulty falling asleep.

5. **Insomnia: Middle of the Night**
   0 = No difficulty.
   1 = Complains of being restless and disturbed during the night.
   2 = Waking during the night—any getting out of bed rates 2 (except for purposes of voiding).

6. **Insomnia: Early Hours of the Morning**
   0 = No difficulty.
   1 = Waking in early hours of the morning, but goes back to sleep.
   2 = Unable to fall asleep again if he/she gets out of bed.

7. **Work and Activities**
   0 = No difficulty.
   1 = Thoughts and feelings of incapacity, fatigue, or weakness related to activities, work, or hobbies.
   2 = Loss of interest in activity, hobbies, or work—either directly reported by patient, or indirectly in listlessness, indecision, and vacillation (feels he/she has to push self to work or activities).
   3 = Decrease in actual time spent in activities or decrease in productivity. Rate 3 if patient does not spend at least 3 hours a day in activities (job or hobbies), excluding routine chores.

8. **Psychomotor Retardation** (slowness of thought and speech, impaired ability to concentrate, decreased motor activity)
   0 = Normal speech and thought.
   1 = Slight retardation during the interview.
   2 = Obvious retardation during the interview.
   3 = Interview difficult.
   4 = Complete stupor.

Continued

Hamilton Depression Rating Scale (HAM-D)—cont'd

4 = Stopped working because of present illness. Rate 4 if patient engages in no activities except routine chores, or if does not perform routine chores unassisted.

9. **Agitation**
   0 = None.
   1 = Fidgetiness.
   2 = Playing with hands, hair, etc.
   3 = Moving about, can't sit still.
   4 = Hand wringing, nail biting, hair pulling, biting of lips.

10. **Anxiety (Psychic)**
    0 = No difficulty.
    1 = Subjective tension and irritability.
    2 = Worrying about minor matters.
    3 = Apprehensive attitude apparent in face or speech.
    4 = Fears expressed without questioning.

11. **Anxiety (Somatic):** Physiological concomitants of anxiety (e.g., dry mouth, indigestion, diarrhea, cramps, belching, palpitations, headache, tremor, hyperventilation, sighing, urinary frequency, sweating, flushing)
    0 = Absent
    1 = Mild.
    2 = Moderate.
    3 = Severe.
    4 = Incapacitating.

12. **Somatic Symptoms (Gastrointestinal)**
    0 = None.
    1 = Loss of appetite, but eating without encouragement. Heavy feelings in abdomen.
    2 = Difficulty eating without urging from others. Requests or requires medication for constipation or gastrointestinal symptoms.

13. **Somatic Symptoms (General)**
    0 = None.
    1 = Heaviness in limbs, back, or head. Backaches, headache, muscle aches. Loss of energy and fatigability.
    2 = Any clear-cut symptom rates 2.

14. **Genital Symptoms** (e.g., loss of libido, impaired sexual performance, menstrual disturbances)
    0 = Absent.
    1 = Mild.
    2 = Severe.

Continued

Hamilton Depression Rating Scale (HAM-D)—cont'd

15. **Hypochondriasis**
    0 = Not present.
    1 = Self-absorption (bodily).
    2 = Preoccupation with health.
    3 = Frequent complaints, requests for help, etc.
    4 = Hypochondriacal delusions.

17. **Insight**
    0 = Acknowledges being depressed and ill.
    1 = Acknowledges illness but attributes cause to bad food, climate, overwork, virus, need for rest, etc.
    2 = Denies being ill at all.

16. **Loss of Weight (Rate *either* A *or* B)**
    A. According to subjective patient history:
    0 = No weight loss.
    1 = Probably weight loss associated with present illness.
    2 = Definite weight loss associated with present illness.
    B. According to objective weekly measurements:
    0 = Less than 1 lb. weight loss in week.
    1 = Greater than 1 lb. weight loss in week.
    2 = Greater than 2 lb. weight loss in week.

TOTAL SCORE _____

Scoring:
0–7 = Normal
8–13 = Mild Depression
14–18 = Moderate Depression
19–22 = Severe Depression
≥23 = Very Severe Depression

From Hamilton, M. (1960). A rating scale for depression. *Journal of Neurology, Neurosurgery, & Psychiatry*, 23: 56-62. In the public domain.

Hamilton Anxiety Rating Scale (HAM-A)

Below are descriptions of symptoms commonly associated with anxiety. Assign the client the rating between 0 and 4 (for each of the 14 items) that best describes the extent to which he/she has these symptoms.

0 = Not present   1 = Mild   2 = Moderate   3 = Severe   4 = Very severe

Rating	Rating
1. **Anxious mood** ——————— Worries, anticipation of the worst, fearful anticipation, irritability	2. **Tension** ——————— Feelings of tension, fatigability, startle response, moved to tears easily, trembling, feelings of restlessness, inability to relax
3. **Fears** ——————— Of dark, of strangers, of being left alone, of animals, of traffic, of crowds	4. **Insomnia** ——————— Difficulty in falling asleep, broken sleep, unsatisfying sleep and fatigue on waking, dreams, nightmares, night terrors
5. **Intellectual** ——————— Difficulty in concentration, poor memory	6. **Depressed mood** ——————— Loss of interest, lack of pleasure in hobbies, depression, early waking, diurnal swing
7. **Somatic (muscular)** ——————— Pains and aches, twitching, stiffness, myoclonic jerks, grinding of teeth, unsteady voice, increased muscular tone	8. **Somatic (sensory)** ——————— Tinnitus, blurred vision, hot/cold flushes, feelings of weakness, tingling sensation
9. **Cardiovascular symptoms** ——————— Tachycardia, palpitations, pain in chest, throbbing of vessels, feeling faint	10. **Respiratory symptoms** ——————— Pressure or constriction in chest, choking feelings, sighing, dyspnea

Continued

Continued

Hamilton Anxiety Rating Scale (HAM-A)—cont'd

11. Gastrointestinal symptoms	12. Genitourinary symptoms
Difficulty swallowing, flatulence, abdominal pain and fullness, burning sensations, nausea/vomiting, borborygmi, diarrhea, constipation, weight loss	Urinary frequency, urinary urgency, amenorrhea, menorrhagia, loss of libido, premature ejaculation, impotence

13. Autonomic symptoms	14. Behavior at interview
Dry mouth, flushing, pallor, tendency to sweat, giddiness, tension headache	Fidgeting, restlessness or pacing, tremor of hands, furrowed brow, strained face, sighing or rapid respiration, facial pallor, swallowing, clearing throat

Client's Total Score _____

SCORING:

14–17 = Mild Anxiety
18–24 = Moderate Anxiety
25–30 = Severe Anxiety

From Hamilton, M. (1959). The assessment of anxiety states by rating. *British Journal of Medical Psychology, 32*: 50–55.
The HAM-A is in the public domain.

Hoarding Rating Scale

Please use the following scale when answering items below:

0 = No problem
2 = Mild problem (less than weekly) acquires items not needed, or acquires a few unneeded items
4 = Moderate, regularly (once or twice weekly) acquires items not needed, or acquires some unneeded items
6 = Severe, frequently (several times per week) acquires items not needed, or acquires many unneeded items
8 = Extreme, very often (daily) acquires items not needed, or acquires large numbers of unneeded items

Hoarding Rating Scale—cont'd

1. Because of the clutter or number of possessions, how difficult is it for you to use the rooms in your home?

0	1	2	3	4	5	6	7	8
Not at all Difficult		Mild		Moderate		Severe		Extremely Difficult

2. To what extent do you have difficulty discarding (or recycling, selling, giving away) ordinary things that other people would get rid of?

0	1	2	3	4	5	6	7	8
No Difficulty		Mild		Moderate		Severe		Extreme Difficulty

3. To what extent do you currently have a problem with collecting free things or buying more things than you need or can use or can afford?

0	1	2	3	4	5	6	7	8
None		Mild		Moderate		Severe		Extreme

4. To what extent do you experience emotional distress because of clutter, difficulty discarding, or problems with buying or acquiring things?

0	1	2	3	4	5	6	7	8
None/ Not at all		Mild		Moderate		Severe		Extreme

5. To what extent do you experience impairment in your life (daily routine, job/school, social activities, family activities, financial difficulties) because of clutter, difficulty discarding, or problems with buying or acquiring things?

0	1	2	3	4	5	6	7	8
None/ Not at all		Mild		Moderate		Severe		Extreme

Total Score_____

Interpretation of HRS Total Scores (Tolin et al 2010)

Mean for Nonclinical samples: HRS Total = 3.34; standard deviation = 4.97.

Mean for people with hoarding problems: HRS Total = 24.22; standard deviation = 5.67.

Analysis of sensitivity and specificity suggests an HRS Total clinical cut-off score of 14.

Criteria for Clinically Significant Hoarding: (Tolin et al 2008)

A score of 4 or greater on questions 1 and 2, and a score of 4 or greater on either question 4 or question 5.

Tolin, D.F., Frost, R.O., Steketee, G., Gray, K.D., & Fitch, K.E. (2008). The economic and social burden of compulsive hoarding. *Psychiatry Research, 160*, 200–211.

Tolin, D.F., Frost, R.O., & Steketee, G. (2010). A brief interview for assessing compulsive hoarding: The Hoarding Rating Scale-Interview. *Psychiatry Research, 178*, 147–152, used with permission.

Geriatric Depression Rating Scale (GDS)

Short Version

Choose the best answer for how you have felt over the past week (circle yes or no):

1. Are you basically satisfied with your life? YES/**NO**
2. Have you dropped many of your activities and interests? **YES**/NO
3. Do you feel that your life is empty? **YES**/NO
4. Do you often get bored? **YES**/NO
5. Are you in good spirits most of the time? YES/**NO**
6. Are you afraid that something bad is going to happen to you? **YES**/NO
7. Do you feel happy most of the time? YES/**NO**
8. Do you often feel helpless? **YES**/NO
9. Do you prefer to stay at home, rather than going out and doing new things? **YES**/NO
10. Do you feel you have more problems with memory than most? **YES**/NO
11. Do you think it is wonderful to be alive now? YES/**NO**
12. Do you feel pretty worthless the way you are now? **YES**/NO
13. Do you feel full of energy? YES/**NO**
14. Do you feel that your situation is hopeless? **YES**/NO
15. Do you think that most people are better off than you are? **YES**/NO

Total Score =

Bold answers = depression

GDS Scoring:

12–15 Severe depression

8–11 Moderate depression

5–7 Mild depression

0–4 Normal

(Yesavage et al 1983; Sheikh 1986; GDS Web site: http://www.stanford.edu/~yesavage/)

🚫 **ALERT:** As with all rating scales, further evaluation and monitoring are often needed. Be sure to perform a Mini-Mental State Examination (MMSE) first to screen for/rule out dementia (cognitive deficits).

Mood Disorder Questionnaire

The Mood Disorder Questionnaire (MDQ) is a useful screening tool for bipolar spectrum disorder in an outpatient population. A score of 7 or more yielded a good sensitivity (0.73) and a very good specificity (0.90).

1. Has there ever been a period of time when you were not your usual self (while not using drugs or alcohol) and ...

...you felt so good or so hyper that other people thought you were not your normal self, or you were so hyper that you got into trouble? (circle yes or no for each line, please)	Yes	No
...you were so irritable that you shouted at people or started arguments?	Yes	No
...you felt much more self-confident than usual?	Yes	No
...you got much less sleep than usual and found you didn't really miss it?	Yes	No
...you were much more talkative or spoke faster than usual?	Yes	No
...thoughts raced through your head or you couldn't slow your mind down?	Yes	No
...you were so easily distracted by things around you that you had trouble concentrating or staying on track?	Yes	No
...you had much more energy than usual?	Yes	No
...you were much more active or did many more things than usual?	Yes	No
...you were much more social or outgoing than usual; for example, you telephoned friends in the middle of the night?	Yes	No
...you were much more interested in sex than usual?	Yes	No
...you did things that were unusual for you or that other people might have thought were excessive, foolish, or risky?	Yes	No
...spending money got you or your family into trouble?	Yes	No

Total number of "Yes" responses to question 1

2. If you checked YES to more than one of the above, have several of these ever happened during the **same period of time?**   Yes   No

3. How much of a **problem** did any of these cause you – like being unable to work; having family, money, or legal troubles; getting into arguments or fights?

No problem
Minor problem
Moderate problem
Serious problem

Scoring on following page.

Scoring:

An individual is considered positive for Bipolar Disorder if they answered:

1. "Yes" to at least 7 of the 13 items in question 1 AND
2. "Yes" to question number 2 AND
3. "Moderate" or "Serious" to question number 3.

All three of the criteria should be met. A positive screen indicates that the person should receive a comprehensive diagnostic evaluation for bipolar spectrum disorder by a psychiatrist, licensed psychologist, or advanced practice psychiatric nurse.

From Hirschfeld R, Williams JB, Spitzer RL, et al. Development and validation of a screening instrument for bipolar spectrum disorder: The Mood Disorder Questionnaire. Am J Psychiatry 2000; 157:1873-1875. Reprinted with permission from Dr. Robert MA Hirschfeld.

Suicidal Behaviors Questionnaire-Revised (SBQ-R)

Name _____   Date _____

Instructions: Check the number beside the statement that best applies to you.

1. Have you ever thought about or attempted to kill yourself?
(check one only)

_____ 1. Never.
_____ 2. It was just a brief passing thought.
_____ 3a. I have had a plan at least once to kill myself but did not try to do it.
_____ 3b. I have had a plan at least once and really wanted to die.
_____ 4a. I have attempted to kill myself, but did not want to die.
_____ 4b. I have attempted to kill myself, and really hoped to die.

2. How often have you thought about killing yourself in the past? (check one only)

_____ 1. Never.
_____ 2. Rarely (1 time).
_____ 3. Sometimes (2 times).
_____ 4. Often (3-4 times)
_____ 5. Very Often (5 or more times).

Continued

Suicidal Behaviors Questionnaire-Revised (SBQ-R)—cont'd

3. **Have you ever told someone that you were going to commit suicide, or that you might do it?** (check one only)
   _____ 1. No.
   _____ 2a. Yes, at one time, but did not really want to die.
   _____ 2b. Yes, at one time and really wanted to die.
   _____ 3a. Yes, more than once, but did not want to do it.
   _____ 3b. Yes, more than once and really wanted to do it.

4. **How likely is it you will attempt suicide someday?** (check one only)
   _____ 0. Never   _____ 4. Likely
   _____ 1. No chance at all   _____ 5. Rather likely
   _____ 2. Rather unlikely   _____ 6. Very likely
   _____ 3. Unlikely

SBQ-R Scoring

Item 1: Taps into *lifetime* suicide attempts: suicide ideation and/or suicide attempts:

Selected response 1	Non-suicidal subgroup	1 point
Selected response 2	Suicide risk ideation subgroup	2 points
Selected response 3a or 3b	Suicide plan subgroup	3 points
Selected response 4a or 4b	Suicide attempt subgroup	4 points

Total points =

Item 2: Assesses the *frequency* of suicidal *ideation* over the past 12 months:

Selected response	Never	1 point
Selected response	Rarely (1 time)	2 points
Selected response	Sometimes (2 times)	3 points
Selected response	Often (3–4 times)	4 points
Selected response	Very often (5 or more times)	5 points

Total points =

Scoring continued

Item 3: Taps into the *threat* of suicide *attempt*:

Selected response 1		1 point
Selected response 2a or 2b		2 points
Selected response 3a or 3b		3 points

Total points =

Item 4: Evaluates *self-reported likelihood* of suicidal behavior in the future:

Selected response	Never	0 points
Selected response	No chance at all	1 point
Selected response	Rather unlikely	2 points
Selected response	Unlikely	3 points
Selected response	Likely	4 points
Selected response	Rather likely	5 points
Selected response	Very likely	6 points

Total points =

Total Score =

Sum all the scores checked by respondents.
The total score should range from 3–18.

SBQ-R Explanation

The SBQ-R is a 4 item questionnaire, each item tapping into a different dimension of suicidality.

– Item 1 taps into lifetime suicide ideation and/or suicide attempt.
– Item 2 assesses the frequency of suicidal ideation over the past 12 months.
– Item 3 assesses the threat of suicide attempt.
– Item 4 evaluates self-reported likelihood of suicidal behavior in the future.

Clinical Utility

This very brief, easy to administer questionnaire assesses lifetime ideation, frequency of ideation, threat of suicide, and future likelihood to help identify those at risk for suicide.

Psychometric Properties			
	Cut-off score	Sensitivity	Specificity
Adult general population	≥7	93%	95%
Adult psychiatric population	≥8	80%	91%

SBQ-R from Osman A, Bagge CL, Gutierrez PM, Kinick LC, Kooper BA, Barrios FX. The suicidal behaviors questionnaire-Revised (SBQ-R): Validation with clinical and nonclinical samples. Assessment 2001; 8:443–454, used with permission.

Mini-Mental State Examination (MMSE)

The *Mini-Mental State Examination* is a brief (10-minute) standardized, reliable screening instrument used to assess for cognitive impairment and commonly used to screen for dementia. It evaluates orientation, registration, concentration, language, short-term memory, and visual-spatial aspects and can be scored quickly (24–30 = normal; 18–23 = mild/moderate cognitive impairment; 0–17 = severe cognitive impairment). (Folstein et al 1975; Psychological Assessment Resources, Inc.)

The Clock-Drawing Test

Another test that is said to be possibly more sensitive to *early* dementia is the clock-drawing test. There are many variations and clock is first drawn (by clinician) and divided into tenths or quadrants. Client is asked to put the numbers in the appropriate places and then indicate the time as "ten minutes after eleven." Scoring is based on test used and completion of the tasks (Manos 2012).

Ethnocultural Considerations

With over 400 ethnocultural groups, it is impossible to cover every group within North America. It is important, however, to become familiar with the characteristics and customs of most ethnocultural groups you will be working with and sensitive to any differences.

Ethnicity refers to a common ancestry through which individuals have evolved shared values and customs. This sense of commonality is transmitted over generations by family and reinforced by the surrounding community (McGoldrick, 2005).

Culturally Mediated Beliefs and Practices

	Dying/birth	Role Differences	Religion	Communication
African American	Reluctant to donate organs. Ask about advance directives/durable power of attorney (may not have any) – usually family makes decisions as a whole. Burials may take up to 5–7 d after death. Varied responses to death.	Varies by educational level/socioeconomic level. High percentage of families is matriarchal. Extended family important in health education; include women in decision making/health information.	Baptist/Methodist/other Protestant/Muslim (Nation of Islam/other sects) Determine affiliation during interview/determine importance of church/religion.	*Eye Contact:* Demonstrates respect/trust, but direct contact may be interpreted as aggressive. *Other:* Silence may indicate distrust. Prefer use of last name (upon greeting) unless referred to otherwise.
Arab American	Colostrum is believed harmful to the infant Death is God's will; turn patient's bed to face Mecca and read the Koran. No cremation, no autopsy (except forensic) and organ donation acceptable.	Men make most decisions (patrilineal) and women responsible for daily needs (wield a lot of influence over family and home); family loyalty more important than individual needs.	Muslim (usually Sunni)/Protestant/Greek orthodox/other Christian. Duties of Islam: Declaration of faith, prayer 5 times/d, alms-giving, fasting during Ramadan, and pilgrimage to Mecca.	*Eye Contact:* Females may avoid eye contact with males/strangers. *Other:* Supportive family members may need a break from caregiving; obtain an interpreter if necessary.

Continued

Culturally Mediated Beliefs and Practices—cont'd

	Dying/birth	Role Differences	Religion	Communication
Asian American	May use incense/ spiritual. Need extra time with deceased members; natural cycle of life.	Father/eldest son primary decision maker; recognized head has great authority.	Primarily Buddhism and Catholicism; Taoism and Islam.	*Eye Contact:* Direct eye contact may be viewed as disrespectful. *Other:* Use interpreters whenever possible (be careful about tone of voice). Often a formal distance.
Native Americans	Full family involvement throughout life cycle; do not practice birth control or limit size of family.	Varies tribe to tribe; most tribes matrilineal and be gate-keeper of the tribe.	Traditional Native American or Christian; spirituality based on harmony with nature.	*Eye Contact:* Eye contact sustained. *Other:* American Ind an may be term preferred by older adults; use an interpreter to avoid misunderstandings. Do not point with finger.

Continued

Culturally Mediated Beliefs and Practices—cont'd

	Dying/birth	Role Differences	Religion	Communication
Mexican Americans	Family support during labor; very expressive during bereavement (find a place where family can grieve together quietly). Fertility practices follow Catholic teachings. Abortion considered wrong.	Equal decision making with all family members; men expected to provide financial support.	Roman Catholic primarily.	*Eye Contact:* Eye contact may be avoided with authority figures. *Other:* Silence may indicate disagreement with proposed plan of care; greet adults formally (señor, señora, etc, unless told otherwise).
Russian Americans	Father may not attend birth; usually closest family female does; family wants to be informed of impending death before patient.	Men and women share decision making; family, women, children highly valued.	Eastern Orthodox and Judaism; remember recent oppression; also Molokans, Tartar Muslims, Pentecostals, Baptists. About 60% not religious.	*Eye Contact:* Direct eye contact acceptable/nodding means approval. *Other:* Use interpreters whenever possible; Russians are distant until trust is established.

Adapted from Purnell & Paulanka 2009 and Myers 2010, with permission

Perception of Mental Health Services: Ethnocultural Differences

African Americans

- Often distrustful of therapy and mental health services. May seek therapy because of child-focused concerns.
- Seek help and support through "the church," which provides a sense of belonging and community (social activities/choir). Therapy is for "crazy people" (McGoldrick 2005).

Mexican Americans

- Understanding the migration of the family is important, including who has been left behind. The church in the barrio often provides community support.
- Curanderos (folk healers) may be consulted for problems such as: mal de ojo (evil eye) and susto (fright) (McGoldrick 2005).

Puerto Ricans

- Nominally Catholic, most value the spirit and soul. Many believe in spirits that protect or harm and the value of incense and candles to ward off the "evil eye."
- Often underutilize mental health services, and therapist needs to understand that expectations about outcome may differ (McGoldrick 2005).

Asian American

- Many Asian-American families are transitioning from the extended family to the nuclear unit and struggling to hold on to old ways while developing new skills.
- Six predictors of mental health problems are: 1) employment/financial status, 2) gender (women more vulnerable), 3) old age, 4) social isolation, 5) recent immigration, and 6) refugee premigration experiences and post-migration adjustment (McGoldrick 2005).

Above are just a few examples of many ethnocultural groups and the differences in the understanding and perception of mental health/therapy.

Culture and the DSM-5

The DSM-5 has taken into consideration culture-specific symptoms, that is, what is considered normal in a specific culture. The challenge for the DSM-5 is aiming for Worldwide applicability of its disorders, when in fact there are cross-cultural variations among disorders. However, the DSM-5 wants culture to be considered in making diagnoses and has developed a Cultural Formulation Interview (CFI). The CFI is a set of 16 questions to be asked during a mental health assessment to determine the impact of culture on patient care (APA 2013; Lewis-Fernandez 2009).

The CFI is located in Section III (Assessment Measures) of the DSM-5 or use following *Ethnocultural* Tool.

Ethnocultural Assessment Tool

Client's name	Ethnic origin
City/State	Birth date
Significant other	Relationship
Primary language spoken	Second language
Interpreter required?	Available?
Highest level of education	Occupation
Presenting problem/chief complaint:	

Have client describe problem "in own words." Has problem occurred before? If so how was it handled?

Client's usual method/s of coping with stress?

Who is (are) client's main support system? Family, friends?

Client's living arrangements (describe):

Major decision maker in family (if applicable):

Client's/family members' roles in the family:

Religious beliefs and practices:

Are there religious restrictions or requirements?

Who takes responsibility for health concerns or problems that arise in family?

Any special concerns or beliefs about client's problem?

Who does client or family usually approach for help/support with problems?

Usual emotional/behavioral response to:

Anger_____

Anxiety_____

Pain_____

Fear_____

Loss/change/failure_____

Sensitive topics client unwilling to discuss due to ethnocultural taboos?

Client's feelings about touch and touching?

Client's feelings regarding eye contact?

Client's orientation to time (past/present/future)?

Illnesses/diseases common to client's ethnicity?

Client's perception of the problem and expectations of care and outcome:

Other:

Modified from Townsend 6th ed., 2014, with permission

Documentation

Problem-Oriented Record (POR)		
POR	**Data**	**Nursing Process**
S (Subjective)	Client's verbal reports (e.g., "I feel nervous")	Assessment
O (Objective)	Observation (e.g., client is pacing)	Assessment
A (Assessment)	Evaluation/interpretation of S and O	Diagnosis/outcome identification
P (Plan)	Actions to resolve problem	Planning
I (Intervention)	Descriptions of actions completed	Implementation
E (Evaluation)	Reassessment to determine results and necessity of new plan of action	Evaluation

Focus Charting (DAR)

Charting	Data	Nursing Process
D (Data)	Describes observations about client/supports the stated focus	Assessment
Focus	Current client concern/behavior/significant change in client status	Diagnosis/outcome identification
A (Action)	Immediate/future actions	Plan and implementation
R (Response)	Client's response to care or therapy	Evaluation

PIE Method (APIE)

Charting	Data	Nursing Process
A (Assessment)	Subjective and objective data collected at each shift	Assessment
P (Problem)	Problems being addressed from written problem list and identified outcomes	Diagnosis/outcome identification
I (Intervention)	Actions performed directed at problem resolution	Plan and implementation
E (Evaluation)	Response appraisal to determine intervention effectiveness	Evaluation

POR, DAR, and APIE modified from Townsend 6th ed., 2014, with permission

CLINICAL PEARL: It is important to systematically assess and evaluate all clients and to develop a plan of action, reevaluating all outcomes. It is equally important to document all assessments, plans, treatments, and outcomes. You may "know" you provided competent treatment, but without documentation there is *no record* from a legal perspective. *Do not ever become complacent about documentation.*

Example of APIE Charting

DATE/TIME	PROBLEM	PROGRESS NOTE
5-22-13 1000	Social isolation	A: States he does not want to sit with or talk to others; they "frighten him." Stays in room; no social involvement. P: Social isolation due to inability to trust. I: Spent time alone with client to initiate trust; accompanied client to group activities; praised participation. E: Cooperative although still uncomfortable in presence of group; accepted positive feedback.

Example modified from Townsend 8th ed., 2014, with permission

Psychiatric Disorders/Interventions

Psychiatric Disorders

Psychiatric Interventions

Neurocognitive Disorders

Previously classified under *Delirium, Dementia, Amnestic, and Other Cognitive Disorders* in the DSM-IV-TR (APA 2000). These disorders are characterized by clinically significant cognitive deficits and notable changes from previous levels of functioning. Neurocognitive disorders will be classified as mild or major based on the severity of the symptoms. Deficits may also be due to a medical condition or substance use or both (APA 2013).

■ Many *Neurocognitive Disorders* are characterized *by intellectual decline and usually progressive deficits* not only in memory, but also in language, perception, learning, and other areas.
■ *Neurocognitive Disorder due to Alzheimer's Disease* (AD) is the most common neurocognitive disorder, followed by *Vascular Neurocognitive Disorder.*
■ *Other causes*: Infections: HIV, encephalitis, Creutzfeldt-Jakob disease; drugs and alcohol (Wernicke-Korsakoff syndrome [thiamine deficiency]); inherited, such as Parkinson's disease and Huntington's disease. Some neurocognitive disorders (AD) are essentially irreversible, and others are potentially reversible (drug toxicities, folate deficiency).

DSM-5 Neurocognitive Disorders

■ Delirium
  ■ Other Specified Delirium
  ■ Unspecified Delirium
■ Mild Neurocognitive Disorder
■ Major Neurocognitive Disorder
■ Subtypes of Major and Mild Neurocognitive Disorders
  ■ Neurocognitive Disorder due to Alzheimer's Disease
  ■ Vascular Neurocognitive Disorder
  ■ Frontotemporal Neurocognitive Disorder (previously Pick's Disease)
  ■ Neurocognitive Disorder due to Traumatic Brain Injury
  ■ Neurocognitive Disorder With Lewy Bodies
  ■ Neurocognitive Disorder due to Parkinson's Disease
  ■ Neurocognitive Disorder due to HIV Infection
  ■ Substance/Medication-Induced Neurocognitive Disorder
  ■ Neurocognitive Disorder due to Huntington's Disease
  ■ Neurocognitive Disorder due to Prion Disease (e.g., Creutzfeldt-Jakob disease)

- Neurocognitive Disorder due to Another Medical Condition (e.g., thiamine deficiency, MS)
- Unspecified Neurocognitive Disorder

(APA 2013) (See full listing of disorders in *Tools* Tab.)

Mild Neurocognitive Disorder

Cognitive decline is modest from previous level of performance with no loss of independence, although support may be needed to retain independence (APA 2013).

Major Neurocognitive Disorder

Cognitive decline is substantial from previous level of performance; requires help with ADLs/paying bills (APA 2013).

Delirium

Organic brain syndrome resulting in a *disturbance in consciousness and cognition that happens within a short period,* with a variable course.

Pseudodementia

Cognitive difficulty that is caused by depression, but may be mistaken for neurocognitive disorder (e.g., AD). Need to consider and rule out depression in the elderly, who may appear to have some form of neurocognitive disorder, when actually suffering from a treatable depression. However, could be depressed with cognitive deficits as well.

CLINICAL PEARL: AD is a *progressive and irreversible disorder* with a gradually declining course, whereas *vascular neurocognitive disorder* (ministrokes and transient ischemic attacks) often presents in a *stepwise fashion,* with an acute decline in cognitive function. It is important to distinguish between the different types of neurocognitive disorder (AD vs. delirium) because delirium can be life-threatening and should be viewed as an emergency. Delirium can be differentiated from other neurocognitive disorders by its *rapid onset, fluctuating in and out of a confusional state, and difficulty in attending to surroundings.* Delirium is usually caused by a physical condition, such as infection (e.g., urinary tract infection); therefore, the underlying cause needs to be treated. Keep in mind that a person with dementia may also become delirious.

Neurocognitive Disorder due to Alzheimer's Disease (AD)

Signs & Symptoms	Causes	Rule Outs	Labs/Tests/Exams	Interventions
• Cognitive impairment/ memory impairment • Inability to learn new material • Language deterioration (naming objects) • Inability to execute typical tasks (cook/ dress self) • Executive functioning disturbances (planning/ abstract thinking/new tasks) • Paranoia • Progressive from mild forgetfulness to moderate to severe cognitive decline & total ADL care/ bedridden • Course: 18 mo–27 y [avg. 10–12 y]	• Idiopathic • Many theories (viral/trauma) • Pathology shows amyloid plaques and neurofibrillary tangles; also amyloid protein (Delrieu 2012) • Familial AD (presenilin 1 gene) • Neuroinflammation (Ferretti 2012) • Apolipoprotein E genotype (Yildiz 2012)	• Vascular neurocognitive disorder • Dementia with Lewy bodies • Alcohol-induced (Wernicke-Korsakoff [thiamine deficiency]; pellagra [niacin deficiency]; hepatic encephalitis) • Delirium • Depression • Medical disorder (HIV, syphilis) • Other: substance-induced • Psychosis	• Mental status exam • Folstein Mini-Mental State Exam • Neuropsychological testing (Boston naming; Wisconsin card sorting test) • Depression Rating Scales; HAM-D; Beck (BDI); Geriatric Depression Scale • CSC, blood chemistry (renal, metabolic/hepatic), sed rate, T4/TSH, B_{12}, folate, U/A, FTA-Abs, CT scan/MRI; HIV titer • Structural MRIs and CSF markers (Andersson 2011; Vemuri 2010) • 18F-FDG positron emission tomography (Bohnen 2012)	• Early diagnosis (mild impairment) • S/mptom treatment: aggression/agitation • Behavioral management • Communication techniques • Environmental safety checks • Antipsychotics (caution) • Assist/perform ADLs • Antidepressants • Sedatives • Antianxiety agents • Nutritional support • Anti-Alzheimer's agents, e.g., donepezil (Aricept); memantine (Namenda) • Molecular novel treatments (HQSAR) (de Souza 2012) • Immunotherapy (Delrieu 2012)

Neurocognitive Disorder With Lewy Bodies

Clients with Lewy body disease usually present with pronounced changes in attention (drowsiness, staring), parkinsonian symptoms, and visual hallucinations. Unlike AD, the course is usually rapid. Researchers are exploring newer methods for diagnosing and differentiating the neurocognitive disorders, including CSF biomarkers (Andersson 2011) and structural MRI (Vernuri 2010).

⊘ **ALERT:** Important to differentiate AD from Lewy body disease. Clients with Lewy body disease are very sensitive to antipsychotics, and because of their psychosis (visual hallucinations), they are often treated with an antipsychotic. Such treatment often results in extrapyramidal symptoms (EPS) or worsening of psychotic symptoms (Goroll 2009). Treatments may include cholinesterase inhibitors (e.g., rivastigmine), levodopa, and sometimes quetiapine (Drach 2011).

Neurocognitive Disorders – Early Diagnosis

The Mayo Clinic has developed a framework entitled STAND-Map (STructural Abnormality iNDex) in hopes of diagnosing neurocognitive disorders in living patients. Hopefully from this we will be able to differentiate among AD, Lewy body disease, and frontotemporal lobe degeneration (Mayo Clinic 2009; Vernuri 2010). Fluorodeoxyglucose (^{18}F) positron emission tomography is a useful adjunct, in conjunction with other diagnostic tests, in assessing neurocognitive disorders (Bohnen 2012).

Alzheimer's Disease – Medications

- Medications used to treat mild to moderate AD include tacrine (Cognex), donepezil (Aricept), rivastigmine (Exelon), and galantamine [Reminyl].
- Memantine (Namenda), which is an NMDA receptor antagonist, is approved for treating moderate to severe AD.

Alzheimer's Disease – Advances in Treatments

- Amyloid b (Ab) peptide is an important target for the treatment of AD, with a goal of modifying the disease process. These newer potential treatments are a result of a better understanding of the pathogenesis of AD.
- One of the aims is to clear amyloid plaques in patients with AD, and although there are several new immunological approaches under investigation, these remain hopeful approaches to reversing the pathology of AD (Delrieu 2012).

Neurocognitive Disorders (NCD) – Client/Family Education

- Educate family on how to communicate with loved ones with cognitive impairment, especially if paranoid. Family members should not argue with someone who is agitated or paranoid.

- Focus on positive behaviors, avoiding negative behaviors that do not pose a safety concern.

- Avoid arguments *by talking about how the NCD client is feeling rather than arguing the validity of a statement.* For instance, if the client says that people are coming into the house and stealing, family members can be taught to discuss the feelings around the statement rather than the reality of it ("That must be hard for you, and we will do all we can to keep you safe.").

- Educate family about *environmental safety*, as cognitive impairment clients may forget they have turned on a stove, or they may have problems with balance. Throw rugs may need to be removed and stove disconnected, with family members providing meals.

- Family members need to understand that this is a long-term management issue requiring the *support of multiple health professionals and family and friends.* Management may require medication (e.g., treatment of AD or control of hostility). Medications need to be started at low doses and titrated slowly.

- Keep in mind that a *spouse or family caregiver* is also dealing with his/her own feelings of loss, helplessness, and memories of the person who once was and no longer exists.

- Teach the family caregiver how to manage difficult behaviors and situations in a calm manner, which will help both the family member and the client.

- When there are concerns about a family member wandering off, *GPS tracking systems* are available, as well as more affordable *medical alert bracelets* (such as *www.americanmedical-id.com*), which can be purchased to include an individual's name and a phone number. Or go to *www.alz.org* to access their "medic alert and safe return" program.

- *Caregiver burden.* Remember that the caregiver also needs a break from the day-to-day stress of caring for someone with cognitive impairment. This could involve respite provided by other family members and friends (WebMD Video 2010). Predictors of caregiver burden include hours spent caring, spousal status, gender, and impairments in ADLs (Kim 2012).

Substance-Related and Addictive Disorders

- Substance-Related and Addictive Disorders (previously Substance-Related Disorders [APA 2000]) include disorders related to prescribed medications, alcohol, over-the-counter medications, caffeine, nicotine, steroids, illegal drugs, and others; as well as substances that serve as central nervous system (CNS) stimulants; CNS depressants; and pain relievers; and may alter both mood and behaviors.
- Many substances are accepted by society when used in moderation (alcohol, caffeine); and others are effective in chronic pain management (opioids); but can be abused in some instances and illegal when sold on the street. There are also behavioral addictive disorders to be considered.

Substance Use and Substance-Induced Disorders, Intoxication, and Withdrawal

The classification of Substance Use and Addictive Disorders now includes four groups: 1) Substance Use Disorders (Substance Dependence and Abuse in the DSM-IV-TR [APA 2000]), 2) Substance/Medication-Induced Disorders (located in each specific disorder section), 3) Intoxication, and 4) Withdrawal (APA 2013).

DSM-5 Substance Use and Addictive Disorders

- Substance/Medication-Induced Disorders (see specific disorders; e.g., Anxiety Disorders)
  - Substance/Medication-Induced Psychotic Disorder
  - Substance/Medication-Induced Bipolar Disorder and Related Disorder
  - Substance/Medication-Induced Depressive Disorder
  - Substance/Medication-Induced Anxiety Disorder
  - Substance/Medication-Induced Obsessive-Compulsive and Related Disorder
  - Substance/Medication-Induced Sleep Disorder
  - Substance/Medication-Induced Sexual Dysfunction
  - Substance/Medication-Induced Neurocognitive Disorder
- **Substance-Related Disorders:** Alcohol-Related Disorders
  - Alcohol Use Disorder
  - Alcohol Intoxication
  - Alcohol Withdrawal
  - Other Alcohol-Induced Disorders or Unspecified Alcohol-Related
- Caffeine-Related Disorders
- Cannabis-Related Disorders
- Hallucinogen-Related Disorders
- Inhalant-Related Disorders
- Opioid-Related Disorders

- Sedative-, Hypnotic-, or Anxiolytic-Related Disorders
- Stimulant-Related Disorders
- Tobacco-Related Disorders
- Other (or Unknown) Substance-Related Disorders
- **Non-Substance-Related Disorders:** Gambling Disorder

(APA 2013) (See full listing of disorders in *Tools* Tab.)

Substance-Related Disorders

- *Substance abuse and substance dependence* has been subsumed under each substance use disorder and is no longer listed separately with its own criteria.
- These disorders include alcohol, cannabis, hallucinogen, inhalant, opioid, sedative/hypnotic, stimulant, tobacco, and unknown substance use disorders.
- The criteria for substance abuse in the DSM-IV-TR (2000) included **legal consequences** (such as arrests), but this has been dropped in the DSM-5, as legal requirements for intoxication were too variable and not a reliable criterion.
- **Craving,** which is as a strong desire for a substance (usually specific substance), has been added as a "new diagnostic criterion" for substance use disorder.
- A **Severity Scale** has also been added as follows: 0 or 1 criterion (no diagnosis), 2–3 criteria (mild substance use), 4–5 criteria (moderate), and 6 or more criteria (severe substance use disorder) (APA 2013).

See *Assessment tab* for *Short Michigan Alcohol Screening Test* and *Substance History and Assessment.*

Alcohol Use Disorder
- **Alcohol Use Disorder** (previously *alcohol abuse* and *dependence disorders [DSM-IV-TR 2000]*, now subsumed under *alcohol use disorder*) is a pattern of problematic alcohol use that causes distress and significant impairment. There is a *strong craving* and a *persistent desire to cut down without success*. Eventually impacts social, occupational, and recreational activities. Can result in hazardous activities and continuation in spite of consequences (physical or psychological) and may result in tolerance and/ or withdrawal (APA 2013).

Alcohol Use Disorder

Signs & Symptoms	Causes	Rule Outs	Labs/Tests/Exams	Interventions
• Problematic use of alcohol, same 12-mo period • Intense **cravings** and compulsive use; unsuccessful efforts to cut down • Inordinate time spent obtaining substance or recovering from • Important activities/roles given up • Continue despite physical/psychological problems/physical hazards • **Tolerance** develops: increasingly larger amounts needed for same effect • **Withdrawal symptoms**: uses substance to relieve withdrawal (APA 2013)	• Genetics (hereditary, esp. alcohol) • Biochemical • Psychosocial • Ethnocultural • Need to approach as biopsychosocial disorder • Response to substances can be very individualistic	• Consider comorbidities: mood disorders, such as bipolar/depression. ECA study (Reiger et al 1990): 60.7% diagnosed with bipolar I had lifetime diagnosis of substance use disorders • PTSD: 84% comorbid alcohol/drug problems (Javidi 2012) • Untreated chronic pain • Undiagnosed depression in elderly (isolation a problem)	• SMAST, CAGE questionnaire • AUDIT, Alcohol Screening and Brief Intervention (NIAAA 2012), others • Toxicology screens (emergencies) • HAM-D; Beck Depression Inventory (BDI) (R/O depression) • GDS; MDQ • Labs: Liver function tests (LFTs) – γ-glutamyltransferase (GGT) and mean corpuscular volume (MCV); % CDT (carbohydrate-deficient transferrin) (Anton 2001)	• Early identification, education, and intervention • Confidential and nonjudgmental approach • Evaluate for comorbidities and treat other disorders • Evaluate own attitudes about substance use/dependence • Psychotherapy • Behavior therapy • 12-step programs • Medications: mood stabilizers, antidepressants, naltrexone • Detoxification • Hospitalization

Substance/Medication-Induced Disorders

■ Substance/medication-induced disorders include psychotic disorder, depressive disorder, anxiety disorder, and other substance-induced disorders.

■ Substance/medication-induced symptoms are characteristic of actual diagnostic disorders, but instead are triggered or induced by the medication/substance being used.

Substance Intoxication

■ Recent overuse of a substance, such as an acute alcohol intoxication, that results in a reversible, substance-specific syndrome.

■ Important behavioral (inappropriate behavior) and psychological (alcohol: slurring of speech, poor coordination, impaired memory, stupor, or coma) changes.

■ Can happen with one-time use of substance.

Substance Withdrawal

■ Symptoms (anxiety, irritability, restlessness, insomnia, fatigue) differ and are specific to each substance (cocaine, alcohol). Symptoms develop when a substance is discontinued abruptly after frequent heavy, and prolonged substance use.

Tolerance

■ Using "increasing amounts" of a substance over time to achieve the same effect and markedly diminished effect with continued use (APA 2013).

Substance Addiction and Behavioral Addiction

Substance Addiction

The repeated, compulsive use of a substance that *continues in spite of negative consequences* (physical, social, psychological, etc.). Addiction is most notable when tolerance results in needing increased amounts of the substance, with little effect, and yet there is a *strong craving* for that substance and an inability to stop using the substance, in spite of efforts to do so. Many factors are involved in the predisposition and ultimate use of substances that lead to tolerance and addiction. Factors include genetics (family history), neurobiological influences, psychological (including trauma, PTSD, bipolar disorder, etc.), and cultural influences (group and family attitudes).

Non-Substance-Related Disorders/Behavioral Addiction

Gambling

- Gambling is reclassified from *Impulse-control Disorders Not Elsewhere Classified* (DSM-IV-TR [APA 2000]) to *Substance-Related and Addictive Disorders* (APA 2013). Can be episodic, chronic, or occur only during a specific time in an individual's lifetime.

Gambling Disorder is characterized by the following:

- Persistent need to gamble increasing amounts of money to achieve desired effect, in a 12-month period.
- Cannot control, stop, or cut down on gambling.
- Preoccupied with gambling.
- Irritable, if trying to stop; gambles when distressed.
- Returns to gambling after a loss to repeat behavior.
- Conceals extent of involvement, has lost relationship, job, career, over gambling.
- Turns to others to supply money to continue gambling.
- DSM-5 criteria for gambling disorder, and the severity scale is as follows: mild, 4–5; moderate, 6–7; and severe, all 9 criteria (APA 2013).

Internet Addiction

- Even though there is no evidence or research suggesting Internet addiction exists as a disorder, behaviors can be compulsive, and the Internet offers many opportunities for sexual addicts (DeAngelis 2000; Ng & Weimer-Hastings 2005). The APA will continue to research *Internet Gaming Disorder*, but it will not be listed as a disorder in the DSM-5 and will be placed in section III for conditions that require more research.
- **Pathological Internet Use** is an impulse-control disorder and may correlate with depression, anxiety, ADHD, obsessive-compulsive symptoms, and hostility/aggression. More studies are needed (Carli 2012).

Substance-Related Disorders: Client/Family Education

- Keep in mind that most clients underestimate their substance use (especially alcohol consumption) and that denial is the usual defense mechanism.
- When a substance-related disorder is suspected, it is important to approach the client in a *supportive and nonjudgmental manner*. Focus on the consequences of continued substance use and abuse (physically/emotionally/family/employment), and discuss the need for complete abstinence. Even with a desire to stop, there can be relapses.
- If a substance user will not seek help, then family members should be encouraged to seek help through organizations such as AlAnon (families

of alcoholics) or NarAnon (families of narcotic addicts). AlaTeen is for adolescent children of alcoholics, and Adult Children of Alcoholics (ACOA) is for adults who grew up with alcoholic parents.

■ For problematic substance users, there is Alcoholics Anonymous, Narcotics Anonymous, Overeaters Anonymous, Smokers Anonymous, Women for Sobriety, etc. There is usually a support group available to deal with the unique issues of each addiction.

■ In some instances, medication may be required to manage the withdrawal phase (physical dependence) of a substance. Benzodiazepines may be needed, including inpatient detoxification.

■ Naltrexone, an opioid antagonist, reduces cravings by blocking opioid receptors in the brain and is used in heroin addiction and alcohol addiction (reduces cravings and number of drinking days) (Tai 2004; Rosner 2010).

■ Educate clients and families about the possibility of comorbidities (bipolar disease, chronic pain) and the need to treat these disorders as well.

⊘ **ALERT:** Be aware of the increase in *methamphetamine addiction* in North America, its highly addictive nature, and the devastating social and physical (neurotoxic) consequences of use (Barr et al 2006). Cattie (2012) found elevated neurobehavioral symptoms in chronic methamphetamine users, risking functional decline.

Schizophrenia Spectrum and Other Psychotic Disorders

In 1908, *Eugen Bleuler,* a Swiss psychiatrist, introduced the term *schizophrenia,* which replaced the term *dementia praecox,* used by *Emil Kraepelin* (1896). Kraepelin viewed this disorder as a deteriorating organic disease; Bleuler viewed it as a serious disruption of the mind, a "splitting of the mind." In 1948, *Fromm-Reichman* coined the term *schizophrenogenic mother,* described as cold and domineering, although appearing self-sacrificing. *Bateson* (1973, 1979) introduced the *double bind* theory, wherein the child *could never win* and was always wrong (invalidation disguised as acceptance; illusion of choice; paradoxical communication).

■ Schizophrenia *is a complex disorder,* and it is now accepted that schizophrenia is the result of neurobiological factors rather than due to some early psychological trauma.
  ■ The *lifetime prevalence rate* is about 0.3%–0.7% (APA 2013).
  ■ Onset in the late teens to early 20s, equally affecting men and women.
  ■ Devastating disease for both the client and the family.

- Schizophrenia affects thoughts and emotions to the point that social and occupational functioning is impaired (Susser 2006; Combs 2010).
- About 5%–6% of schizophrenics commit suicide (APA 2013).
- *Early diagnosis and treatment are critical* to slowing the deterioration and decline, which will result without treatment.
- 🚫 **ALERT**: A new blood test, VeriPsych, is available to aid in the diagnosis of schizophrenia. This is a 51-biomarker test that may help with early-onset schizophrenia diagnosis (Schwarz 2010; VeriPsych 2010).
- Earlier typical antipsychotic drugs are effective against most of the positive symptoms; less effective against negative symptoms.
- Atypical antipsychotic drugs work on both negative and positive symptoms.
- Family/community support is key factor in improvement.
- *National Association for the Mentally Ill* (www.nami.org) is an important national organization that has done much to educate society and communities about mental illness and to advocate for the seriously ill.

DSM-5 Schizophrenia Spectrum/Psychotic Disorders

- Brief Psychotic Disorder
- Catatonic Disorder due to Another Medical Condition
- Delusional Disorder
- Psychotic Disorder due to Another Medical Condition
- Schizoaffective Disorder
- Schizophrenia
- Schizophreniform Disorder
- Schizotypal Personality Disorder
- Substance/Medication-Induced Psychotic Disorder
- Other Specified or Unspecified Schizophrenia Spectrum and Other Psychotic Disorder

(APA 2013) (See full listing of disorders in *Tools* Tab.)

Schizophrenia—DSM-5 Changes

DSM-5 has eliminated the special treatment of those with *bizarre delusions/ special hallucinations* and has also removed the *4 subtypes*. Does include a *specifier*: with catatonic features (APA 2013).

- *Subtypes* are no longer considered useful in the clinical setting or for research and have been removed (APA 2013):
  - Paranoid
  - Disorganized
  - Catatonic
  - Undifferentiated
- In DSM-IV-TR (APA 2000), only one criterion (A) was required if the delusions were bizarre (implausible). This no longer applies.
- As with other disorders, the DSM-5 will now focus on *severity* of psychotic signs and symptoms.
- The *Catatonic Specifier* requires 3 or more of the following: 1) cataleptic immobility or stupor; 2) purposeless motor activity; 3) negativity (refusal to change posture) or mutism; 4) posturing, peculiar mannerisms or grimacing; and 5) ecolalia (repeating word/phrase of another person) or ecopraxia (repeating movements of another person) (APA 2013).

Schizophrenia

Signs & Symptoms	Causes	Rule Outs	Labs/Tests/Exams	Interventions
• Usually late adolescence/early adulthood.	• Incidence (US): 0.25–0.50/1,000	• Schizophreniform disorder	• Psychiatric evaluation and mental status exam	• Antipsychotic – usually atypicals: olanzapine, aripiprazole, paliperidone (Invega), etc.
• At least for 1 mo, two or more	• Dopamine hypothesis (excess/glutamate	• Schizoaffective disorder	• No test can diagnose schizophrenia	• New: Adasuve Inhalant (loxapine): agitation in schizophrenia
• Delusions	• Brain: structural abnormalities (third ventricle sometimes larger)	• Mood disorder with psychotic symptoms	• Positive and Negative Syndrome Scale (PANSS)	
• Hallucinations		• Medical disorder/ substance abuse with psychotic episode	• Abnormal Involuntary Movement Scale (AIMS)	• Individual, family, group therapy; social skills training
• Disorganized speech	• Frontal lobe – smaller frontal lobe			
• Abnormal psychomotor behavior	• Genetic – familial; monozygotic twin (47% risk vs. 12% dizygotic)	• Delusional disorder	• Need to R/O other possible medical/ substance use disorders: LFTs,	• Hospitalization until positive symptoms under control
• Negative symptoms (restricted affect, avolition/asociality)	• Prenatal/obstetrical complications	• Note: with schizophrenia, the condition persists for at least 6 mo	toxicology screens, CBC, thyroid function test (TFT), CT scan, etc.	• Program of Assertive Community Treatment (Monroe-DeVita 2012)
• Functional disturbances at school, work, self-care, personal relations	• Winter birth	• Monitor for suicide	• New: VeriPsych blood test (measures 51 biomarkers) (Schwarz 2010; VeriPsych 2010)	• Patient/family education
• Disturbance continues for 6 mo (APA 2013)	• Virus (prenatal as well as childhood)			• NAMI for family, patient advocate
	• No specific cause (Clinical Key 2012)			• The Recovery Model (Warner 2010)

Positive and Negative Symptoms of Schizophrenia

■ *Positive Symptoms*

Positive symptoms are excesses in behavior (excessive function/distortions)

- Delusions
- Hallucinations (auditory/visual)
- Hostility
- Disorganized thinking/behaviors

■ *Negative Symptoms*

Negative symptoms are deficits in behavior (reduced function; self-care deficits)

- Alogia
- Affective blunting
- Anhedonia
- Asociality
- Avolition
- Apathy

Four A's of Schizophrenia

■ Eugen Bleuler in 1911 proposed four basic diagnostic areas for characterizing schizophrenia. These became the 4 A's:

A: Inappropriate **Affect**

A: Loosening of **Associations**

A: **Autistic** thoughts

A: **Ambivalence**

■ These four A's provide a memory tool for recalling how schizophrenia affects thinking, mood (flat), thought processes, and decision-making ability (Shader 2003).

CLINICAL PEARL: When *auditory hallucinations* first begin, they usually sound soft and far away and eventually become louder. When the sounds become soft and distant again, the auditory hallucinations are usually abating. The majority of hallucinations in North America are auditory (versus visual), and it is unlikely that a client will experience both auditory and visual hallucinations at the same time.

Thought Disorders – Content of Thought (Definitions)

Common Delusions

Delusion of Grandeur – Exaggerated/unrealistic sense of importance, power, identity. *Thinks he/she is the President or Jesus Christ.*

Delusion of Persecution – Others are out to harm or persecute in some way. *May believe his/her food is being poisoned or he/she is being watched.*

Delusion of Reference – Everything in the environment is somehow related to the person. *A television news broadcast has a special message for this person solely.*

Somatic Delusion – An unrealistic belief about the body, such as the brain is rotting away.

Control Delusion – Someone or something is controlling the person. *Radio towers are transmitting thoughts and telling person what to do.*

Thought Disorders – Form of Thought (Definitions)

Circumstantiality – Excessive and irrelevant detail in descriptions with the person eventually making his/her point. *We went to a new restaurant. The waiter wore several earrings and seemed to walk with a limp . . . yes, we loved the restaurant.*

Concrete Thinking – Unable to abstract and speaks in concrete, literal terms. *For instance, a rolling stone gathers no moss would be interpreted literally.*

Clang Association – Association of words by sound rather than meaning. *She cried till she died but could not hide from the ride.*

Loose Association – A loose connection between thoughts that are often unrelated. *The bed was unmade. She went down the hill and rolled over to her good side. And the flowers were planted there.*

Tangentiality – Digressions in conversation from topic to topic and the person never makes his/her point. *Went to see Joe the other day. By the way, bought a new car. Mary hasn't been around lately.*

Neologism – Creation of a new word meaningful only to that person. *The hiphopmobility is on its way.*

Word Salad – Combination of words that have no meaning or connection. *Inside outside blue market calling.*

Schizophrenia – Client/Family Education

■ Client and family education is critical to improve chances of relapse prevention and to slow or prevent regression and associated long-term disability.

■ Refer client/family to the National Alliance for the Mentally Ill (NAMI) (www.nami.org) (1-800-950-NAMI [6264]).

- Client needs both medication and family/community support.
- Studies have shown that clients taking medication can still relapse if living with high expressed emotion family members (spouse/parent). These family members are critical, intense, hostile, and overly involved versus low expressed emotion family members (Davies 1994).
- Once stabilized on medication, clients often stop taking their medication *because they feel they no longer need their medication* (denying the illness or believing they have recovered). It is important to stress the need for medication indefinitely and that maintenance medication is needed to prevent relapse.
- Clients also stop their medication because of *untoward side effects.* Engage the client in a discussion about medications so that he/she has some control about options. The newer atypical drugs have a better side-effect profile, but it is important to listen to the client's concerns (weight gain/EPS) as adjustments are possible or a switch to another medication. Educate client/family that periodic lab tests will be needed.

⊘ **ALERT:** For those on antipsychotic therapy, there is also a concern with treatment-emergent diabetes, especially for those with risk factors for diabetes, such as family history, obesity, and glucose intolerance (Buse et al 2002; Smith 2008). (See *Antipsychotics and Treatment Emergent Diabetes* in *Drugs/Labs tab*).

- Early diagnosis, early treatment, and ongoing antipsychotic maintenance therapy with family support are critical factors in slowing the progression of this disease and in keeping those with schizophrenia functional and useful members of society.

Depressive Disorders

Previously classified under *Mood Disorders* (DSM-IV-TR [APA 2000]).

- *Major depressive disorder* (unipolar depression) requires at least 2 weeks of depression/loss of interest and four additional depressive symptoms, with one or more major depressive episodes.
- *Persistent depressive disorder* (dysthymia) is an ongoing low-grade depression of at least 2 years' duration for more days than not and does not meet the criteria for major depression.
- *Unspecified depressive disorder* (previously NOS) does not meet the criteria for major depression and other disorders, including bipolar related disorders (APA 2013).

DSM-5 Depressive Disorders

- Disruptive Mood Dysregulation Disorder
- Persistent Depressive Disorder (Dysthymia)
- Major Depressive Disorder, Recurrent
- Major Depressive Disorder, Single Episode
- Premenstrual Dysphoric Disorder
- Substance/Medication-Induced Depressive Disorder
- Depressive Disorder due to Another Medical Condition
- Other Specified or Unspecified Depressive Disorder

(APA 2013) (See full listing of disorders in *Tools Tab*.)

See *depression rating scales* (HAM-D, Geriatric) in the *Assessment tab* as well as *Suicidal Behaviors Questionnaire-R*.

Disruptive Mood Dysregulation Disorder (DMDD)

- *New disorder* in the DSM-5.
- DMDD added because of concerns of overdiagnosis of bipolar disorder in children.
- Overlapping criteria with oppositional defiant disorder (ODD), but more severe than ODD.
- *Severe recurrent temper outbursts not in proportion to the situation. Verbal and/or physical rages to people or property, 3 or more times a week. Consistently irritable or angry, observable by others, for 12 or more months; ages 7–18 years* (APA 2013). See also ODD, *Intermittent explosive disorder* and *Bipolar disorder*.

Premenstrual Dysphoric Disorder (PDD)

PDD was located in the appendix for further study of DSM-IV-TR (2000) and has now been *added as a new disorder* in the DSM-5.

- 5 or more symptoms most of the time during last week of luteal phase (final week of onset of menses), resolving in the follicular phase.
- Depressed mood, anxiety, mood lability, anger/irritability, decreased interests, lethargy, appetite changes, hypersomnia, insomnia, physical symptoms (bloating, weight gain). Markedly interferes with work, school, relationships (APA 2013).

SIGECAPS – Mnemonic for Depression

Following is a mnemonic for easy recall and review of the DSM-5 criteria for major depression or dysthymia:

Sleep (increase/decrease)
Interest (diminished)
Guilt/low self-esteem
Energy (poor/low)
Concentration (poor)
Appetite (increase/decrease)
Psychomotor (agitation/retardation)
Suicidal ideation
A depressed mood for 2 or more weeks, plus four SIGECAPS = major depressive disorder
A depressed mood, plus three SIGECAPS for 2 years, most days = dysthymia (persistent depressive disorder) (Brigham and Women's Hospital 2001).

CLINICAL PEARL: Important to determine whether a depressive episode is a unipolar depression or a bipolar disorder *with a depressive episode*. A first-episode bipolar disorder may *begin with major depression*. The presentation is a "clinical snapshot in time" rather than the complete picture. Further evaluation and monitoring are needed. Bipolar clients are often misdiagnosed for years.

- One study (Ghaemi et al 2003) showed 37% of patients were misdiagnosed (depression vs. bipolar), resulting in new or worsening rapid cycling (mania) in 23% because antidepressants were prescribed (Keck 2003).
- Although the tricyclic antidepressants (TCAs) are more likely to trigger a manic episode, the selective serotonin reuptake inhibitors (SSRIs) have also been implicated.

⊘ **ALERT:** If a client who has been recently prescribed an antidepressant begins showing manic symptoms, consider that this client may be bipolar.

Postpartum (Peripartum) Major Depressive Episode

- Fifty (50) percent of postpartum depression begins prior to delivery. Mood symptoms begin during pregnancy or in weeks to months following delivery (APA 2013).
- May have severe anxiety, disinterest in the infant, afraid to be with the infant, or overly involved (APA 2013). See *Edinburgh Postnatal Depression Scale* in *Assessment* tab.

Postpartum Depression in Fathers

- Fathers can also develop postpartum depression with a 4%–25% chance. Three to 6 months showed the highest rate (25.6%). Twelve-month prevalence is 4.8% (Melrose 2010).
- Fathers need to be screened for depression, and depression in one parent warrants clinical attention to the other.
- Fathers should also be screened for depression using the EPDS with a cut-off score of over 10 (Edmondson 2010).

Major Depression and the Bereavement Exclusion

In the DSM-IV-TR (APA 2000) there was a *bereavement exclusion criterion* for Major Depressive Disorder that has been eliminated in the DSM-5 (APA 2013). According to the APA, the preponderance of evidence suggests that symptoms related to the loss of a loved one are no different than symptoms related to other losses. There is concern about "pathologizing" normal grief, but the APA (2013) is concerned, given the potential risk for suicide, that those who are suffering from major depression after the loss of a loved one will not qualify for needed treatments and will be left untreated (DSM-5; 2013).

Major Depressive Episode

Signs & Symptoms	Causes	Rule Outs	Labs/Tests/Exams	Interventions
• Depressed mood or loss of interest for 2 weeks; 5 or more of: • Significant weight loss/gain • Insomnia or hypersomnia • Psychomotor agitation or retardation • Fatigue • Worthless feelings or inappropriate guilt • Problem concentrating • Recurrent thoughts of death • **Note:** Removal of grief exclusion (APA 2013)	• Familial predisposition • Deficiency of norepinephrine (NE) and serotonin; also dopamine, GABA • HPA axis dysregulation (Guerry 2011) • Psychosocial factors • Unknown	• Bipolar disorder • Schizoaffective and mental status exam • Postpartum depression • Thyroid/adrenal dysfunction; hypothyroidism • Neoplasms • CNS (stroke) • Vitamin deficiencies (folic acid) • Medication (reserpine, prednisone) • Pseudodementia (older adult) • Substance use • Monitor for suicide	• Psychiatric evaluation and mental status exam • HAM-D; BDI; Zung Self-Rating Depression Scale; Geriatric Depression Scale • Mood Disorder Questionnaire • Suicidal Behaviors Questionnaire • EEG abnormalities • MMSE • Physical exam • Dexamethasone suppression test • R/O other possible medical/substance use disorders: LFTs, toxicology screens, CBC, TFT, CT scan, etc.	• Antidepressants: usually SSRIs (fluoxetine, sertraline); selective norepinephrine reuptake inhibitors (SNRIs) (venlafaxine) • TCAs; side effects include sedation, dry mouth, blurred vision; TCAs not good for elderly (falls) • MAOIs • Selegiline patch (Emsam) • Others: bupropion • Cognitive behavioral therapy (CBT) • Psychotherapy • Electroconvulsive therapy (ECT) • Vagal nerve stimulation • Transcranial magnetic stimulation

Postpartum (Peripartum) Major Depressive Episode

Signs & Symptoms	Causes	Rule Outs	Labs/Tests/Exams	Interventions
• Symptoms similar to major depressive episode • Acute onset to slowly over first 3 months postpartum (PP), can start in pregnancy • Persistent/ debilitating vs. blues • Depressed mood, tearfulness, insomnia, suicidal thoughts • Anxiety, obsession about well-being of infant • Affects functioning (APA 2013)	• Occurs in 10%–15% of women and 4%–25% of men • Highest risk: hx of depression, previous PP depression, depression during pregnancy • Previous PP depression with psychosis: ↑30%–50% risk of recurrence at subsequent delivery (APA 2013)	• PP "baby" blues (fluctuating mood; peaks 4th d post delivery; ends 2 weeks; functioning intact) • PP psychosis: 1 in 500/1000 deliveries ↑ risk: bipolar/previous PP psychosis; infanticide/suicide risk high (APA 2013) • Medical cause	• Edinburgh Postnatal Depression Scale (EPDS): self-rated questionnaire and Suicidal Behaviors Questionnaire-R (see *Assessment tab*); also to screen fathers • Screen during PP period • Psychiatric evaluation • Physical exam • Routine lab tests: CBC, TFT (thyroid/anemia)	• Pharmacological: SSRIs, SNRIs, TCAs (insomnia); consider weight gain, dry mouth, sedation with TCAs • CBT, individual, group psychotherapy • Family support; also support father • Anxiolytics • ECT • Psychosis: hospitalization; mood stabilizers, antipsychotics, ECT

Bipolar and Related Disorders

Previously classified under *Mood Disorders* (DSM-IV-TR [APA 2000]).

- *Bipolar I disorder* includes one or more manic or mixed episodes, usually with a major depressive episode.
- *Bipolar II disorder* includes one or two major depressive episodes and at least one hypomanic (less than full mania) episode.
- *Cyclothymic disorder* includes at least 2 years of hypomanic/depressive periods that do not meet the full criteria for other disorders.
- *Others:* Bipolar disorder due to another medical condition, substance/ medication-induced bipolar disorder, and other or unspecified bipolar and related disorder (APA 2013).

See the *Mood Disorder Questionnaire (MDQ) (Hirschfeld 2003)* for bipolar spectrum disorder in the *Assessment tab;* also *Suicidal Behaviors Questionnaire-R.*

DSM-5 Bipolar Disorders

- Bipolar I Disorder
- Bipolar II Disorder
- Cyclothymic Disorder
- Substance/Medication-Induced Bipolar and Related Disorders
- Bipolar and Related Disorder due to Another Medical Condition
- Other Specified or Unspecified Bipolar and Related Disorder

(APA 2013) (See full listing of disorders in *Tools* Tab.)

Manic Episode

Signs & Symptoms	Causes	Rule Outs	Labs/Tests/Exams	Interventions
• Persistent elevated, irritable mood ≥1 wk, plus three or more (irritable, four or more): • ↑ Self-esteem • ↓ Sleep • ↑ Talk/pressured speech • Racing thoughts/ flight of ideas • Distractibility • Extreme goal-directed activity • Excessive buying/sex/ business investments (painful consequences) (APA 2013)	• Genetic: familial predisposition (female-to-male, 1.1:1) • Lifetime US prevalence Bipolar I: 0.6% (APA 2013) • Bipolar onset 18–20 y • Catecholamines: NE, dopamine • Many hypotheses: serotonin, acetylcholine; neuroanatomical (frontotemporal lesions) • Complex disorder	• Hypomanic episode (bipolar II) • Anxiety disorder • Cyclothymia • Substance-induced (cocaine) • ADHD • Dual diagnosis • Brain lesion • General medical condition • Monitor for suicide for bipolar clients in depressive phase ~ 10%–15% bipolar I clients complete suicide	• Psychiatric evaluation and mental status exam • Young Mania Rating Scale (YMRS) (bipolar I) • Mood Disorder Questionnaire • Need to R/O other possible medical/ substance use/ induced disorders: LFTs, toxicology screens, CBC, TFT, CT scan, etc.	• Mood stabilizers: lithium, carbamazepine, valproic acid, lamotrigine, topiramate • Combined: lithium and anticonvulsant • Antipsychotics: e.g., aripiprazole, olanzapine • Lithium: + for mania/ not for mixed • *New*: Bipolar I agitation: Adasuve Inhalant (loxapine) (acute mania) • Hospitalization • Individual, family therapy and medication adherence

Depressive and Bipolar Disorders – Client/Family Education

Family and client need educating about the specific disorder, whether major depression, bipolar I or II, or postpartum depression. Without treatment, support, and education, the results can be devastating emotionally, interpersonally, legally, and financially.

- These disorders need to be explained in terms of their *biochemical basis* – "depression is an illness, not a weakness," although often a recurrent, chronic illness.
- Families and clients need to understand that *early diagnosis and treatment* are essential for effective management and improved outcome.
- It may be helpful to compare with other chronic illnesses, such as diabetes and asthma, as a model and to *reinforce the biological basis of the illness* to reduce stigma. As with any chronic illness, ongoing management, including pharmacological treatment, is required, realizing there may be exacerbations and remissions.
- Reinforce the need to *adhere to the dosing schedule as prescribed* and not to make any unilateral decisions, including stopping medications, without conferring with health professional.
- Work with client and family on *side-effect management. If client can be part of the decision making* when there are options, client will be more willing to become involved in own recovery and continue treatment.
- *Address weight gain possibilities* (lithium, anticonvulsants, antipsychotics); monitor weight, BMI, exercise, and food plans to prevent weight gain.
- *Other treatment options for depression*: Mindfulness, CBT, and transcranial magnetic stimulation; also exercise (Segal 2010; George 2010).

Anxiety Disorders

- The *anxiety disorders* include a wide range of disorders from the very specific, such as phobias, to generalized anxiety disorder, which is pervasive and experienced as dread or apprehension.
- Some anxiety is good, motivating people to perform at their best. Excessive anxiety can be crippling and may result in the "fight or flight" reaction. The fighter is ever ready for some perceived aggression and is unable to relax, and the escaper (flight) freezes with anxiety and may avoid upsetting situations or actually dissociate (leave his/her body/fragment).
- Either extreme is not good and can result in physical and emotional exhaustion. (See *Fight-or-Flight Response* and *Stress-Adaptation Syndrome* in *Basics* tab.)

Four Levels of Anxiety

- *Mild anxiety* – This is the anxiety that can motivate someone positively to perform at a high level. It helps a person to focus on the situation at hand. For instance, this kind of anxiety is often experienced by performers before entering the stage.
- *Moderate anxiety* – Anxiety moves up a notch with narrowing of the perceptual field. The person has trouble attending to his/her surroundings, although he/she can follow commands/direction.
- *Severe anxiety* – Increasing anxiety brings the person to another level, resulting in an inability to attend to his/her surroundings except for maybe a detail. Physical symptoms may develop, such as sweating and palpitations (pounding heart). Anxiety relief is the goal.
- *Panic anxiety* – The level reached is now terror, where the only concern is to escape. Communication impossible at this point (Peplau 1963).

CLINICAL PEARL: Recognizing level of anxiety is important in determining intervention. Important to manage anxiety *before it escalates.* At the moderate level, firm, short, direct commands are needed: *You need to sit down, Mr. Jones.*

DSM-5 Anxiety Disorders

- Generalized Anxiety Disorder
- Agoraphobia
- Panic Disorder*
- Separation Anxiety Disorder
- Social Anxiety Disorder (Social Phobia)
- Specific Phobia
- Substance/Medication-Induced Anxiety Disorder
- Anxiety Disorder due to Another Medical Condition
- Other Specified or Unspecified Anxiety Disorder
- Panic Disorder. (See full listing of disorders in *Tools Tab*.)

*Panic disorder is no longer listed as "with or without agoraphobia." These are now treated as two separate disorders in the DSM-5 (APA 2013).

Separation Anxiety Disorder

In the DSM-IV-TR (2000), there was an early-onset specifier (6 y), and onset was before age 18. There are no such specifiers or criteria for DSM-5 (2013). This was previously classified under *Other Disorders of Infancy, Childhood, or Adolescence* (APA 2000).

- Excessive fear concerning separation and developmentally inappropriate – from an attachment figure or home. At least 3 criteria:
  - Recurrent distress over leaving home or attachment figure, excessive worry about loss of figure, refusal to leave home, fear of being alone, refusal to sleep away from home or figure, nightmares with separation themes and physical symptoms, with anxiety lasting 4 weeks in children/adolescents and 6 months or more in adults. (APA 2013).

Generalized Anxiety Disorder

- Excessive anxiety that is difficult to control. Worried about future events.
- A diagnosis for GAD requires excessive anxiety for at least 6 months. (APA 2013).
- Other anxiety disorders include separation anxiety disorder, panic disorder, agoraphobia (avoidance of places that may result in panic), social anxiety disorder (social phobia), specific phobia, selective mutism, anxiety due to another medical condition, substance/medication-induced anxiety disorder, and other disorders.

(See the *Hamilton Anxiety Rating Scale* in the *Assessment* Tab.)

Generalized Anxiety Disorder (GAD)

Signs & Symptoms	Causes	Rule Outs	Labs/Tests/Exams	Interventions
• Excessive anxiety; at least 6 mo; difficult to control worry/hypervigilant • Associated with three or more: • Restless/on edge • Easily fatigued • Concentration problems • Irritability • Muscle tension • Sleep disturbance • Causes significant distress • Often physical complaints: dizziness, tachycardia, tightness of chest, sweating, tremor (APA 2013)	• Neurotransmitter dysregulation: NE, 5-HT, GABA • Autonomic nervous system activation: locus ceruleus/NE release/limbic system • 1-year prevalence rate: 2.9%; (APA 2013) • Familial association • Over half: onset in childhood	• Anxiety disorder due to medical condition (hyperthyroidism; pheochromocytoma) • Substance-induced anxiety or caffeine-induced anxiety disorder • Other disorders: panic disorder, OCD, PTSD, social anxiety disorder, etc. • Anxiety and depression often co-occur.	• Self-rated scales: Beck Anxiety Inventory (BAI); State Trait Anxiety Inventory • Observer-rated scale: Hamilton Anxiety Rating Scale (HAM-A) (See Assessment Tab); depression scales (HAM-D) • Psychiatric evaluation • Physical exam • Routine lab tests; TFTs	• Pharmacological: benzodiazepines very effective (diazepam, lorazepam); nonbenzodiazepines: buspirone • Antidepressants, (SSRIs): escitalopram and paroxetine • Beta blockers: propranolol • CBT/mindfulness CBT • Meditation • Deep muscle relaxation • Individual and family therapy • Education

Client/Family Education – Anxiety Disorders

Anxiety, the most common disorder in the United States, exists along a continuum and may be in response to a specific stressor (taking a test), or it may present as a generalized "free-floating" anxiety (GAD) or a panic disorder (PD) (feeling of terror). A 1-year prevalence rate for all anxieties has been said to be about 18.1% (NIMH 2010).

- Most people have experienced some degree of anxiety, so it might be helpful for family members to understand the four stages of anxiety and how one stage builds on the other – especially in trying to explain panic disorder.
- It is important for families to understand the importance of *early diagnosis and treatment* of anxiety disorders because these are chronic illnesses and will become worse and more difficult to treat over time.
- Explain to client and family the need for *ongoing management* (pharmacological/education/psychotherapeutic/CBT/mindfulness CBT), just as diabetes, asthma, and heart disease must be managed.
- *Stress reduction* through exercise, meditation, biofeedback, and mindfulness CBT can help with reducing anxiety.
- *Medication management* can prove very helpful, such as benzodiazepines for management of acute or situational anxiety or panic disorder. (Increased risk of physical/psychological dependence with long-term use.) SSRIs are also very helpful in treating anxiety, such as paroxetine, which has been used for panic disorder, social anxiety, and generalized anxiety disorders.
- The client may also need to *be educated about the needs of other family members* (maybe time away from client [respite]). Family therapy may be needed to negotiate and agree on living arrangements in a way that respects the needs of the client and all family members.
- Remind families that *patience, persistence*, and a *multimodal/multi-team approach* to treatment are needed.

Obsessive-Compulsive and Related Disorders

This is a new classification in the DSM-5 (APA 2013) and was part of the *Anxiety Disorders* in DSM-IV-TR (APA 2000).

DSM-5 Obsessive-Compulsive and Related Disorders

- Body Dysmorphic Disorder
- Excoriation (Skin-Picking) Disorder (*New to DSM-5*)

- Trichotillomania (Hair-Pulling Disorder)
- Hoarding Disorder
- Obsessive-Compulsive Disorder
- Substance/Medication-Induced Obsessive-Compulsive and Related Disorders
- Obsessive-Compulsive and Related Disorder due to Another Medical Condition
- Other Specified or Unspecified Obsessive-Compulsive and Related Disorder (APA 2013) (See full listing of disorders in *Tools Tab*)

Obsessive Compulsive Disorder (OCD)

- Individuals with OCD are plagued by time-consuming, persistent *obsessions* and *compulsions* to perform certain repetitive actions to reduce anxiety. Obsessions may include a fear of contamination believing horrible consequences if certain rituals aren't performed. Rituals can include repetitive hand washing or having to turn a light switch on and off multiple times, until the anxiety is reduced (APA 2013).
- Both *pharmacological* (e.g., fluoxetine) and *behavioral treatments* (CBT) have proven successful in at least managing symptoms and reducing stress and the need to perform these rituals.

Hoarding Disorder

- *New disorder in the DSM-5.*
- Occurs in 2%–5% of the population and leads to substantial distress (Mataix-Cols 2010) and warrants own diagnosis in DSM-5 (Timpano 2011).
- Difficulty letting go of possessions and discarding even if of little value; living space becomes cluttered resulting in congestion; impairs social, work, and interpersonal areas of life; and environment becomes unsafe and a public health hazard.
- Functional MRIs of the brain demonstrated abnormal activity in the *anterior cingulate cortex and insula*, which showed *excessive activity when having to make decisions about discarding personal possessions.* These brain areas were not affected by items not belonging to the participants, but were activated by personal items that then resulted in the inability to make a decision about discarding. Neural function activity correlated significantly with severity of hoarding and self-ratings of indecisiveness (Tolin 2012).
- Should not be part of another disorder such as obsessions in OCD or major depression (reduced energy). Need to specify if hoarding is excessive as well as degree of insight (APA 2013).
- Hoarding disorder can be difficult to treat and has genetic and neurobiological underpinnings. Inability to let go of items relates to belief systems and emotional ties and linking to items.

- Treatments include the use of SSRIs, adjunctive medications such as antipsychotics and mood stabilizers, as well as cognitive behavioral treatment. SSRIs may also treat comorbid disorders such as OCD and depression. Insight and motivation, as well as family support, important for change to take place. SSRIs plus CBT likely more effective (Feusner 2005; Saxena 2011). (See *Hoarding Rating Scale* in *Assessment tab*.)

Body Dysmorphic Disorder

- *Body Dysmorphic Disorder* previously under *Somatoform Disorders* (DSM-IV-TR [APA 2000]).
- *Body Dysmorphic Disorder* (BDD) is an obsession/preoccupation with an (perceived) exaggerated "defect" (nose, lips, eyes) in physical appearance, with frequent checking in the mirror. Preoccupation causes significant distress and social, occupational, or other functional impairment. DSM-5 (APA 2013) views this as a condition belonging in the OCD classification of disorders.

Tricotillomania

- *Tricotillomania* (hair-pulling disorder) previously classified under *Impulse Control Disorders* (DSM-IV-TR [APA 2000]).
- *Tricotillomania* is the recurrent and compulsive pulling out of hair, causing distress, but with an inability to stop. May impair work, social, and other areas of functioning (APA 2013).

Obsessive-Compulsive Disorder (OCD)

Signs & Symptoms	Causes	Rule Outs	Labs/Tests/Exams	Interventions
• Usually starts in adolescence/early adulthood • *Obsessions* – recurrent, intrusive thoughts that cause anxiety OR *Compulsions* – repetitive behaviors (hand washing, checking) that reduce distress/anxiety and must be adhered to rigidly • Driven to perform compulsions • Time-consuming (>1 hr/d), interferes with normal routine • May have absent to good insight (APA 2013)	• Genetic evidence • Neurobiological basis: orbitofrontal cortex, cingulate, and caudate nucleus • Neurochemical: serotoninergic and possibly dopaminergic • Association between OCD and Tourette's, and others • 12-month US prevalence of 1.2% • Early onset: 6–15 y (usually males) • Adult onset: 20–29 y (usually female) (APA 2013)	• Other disorders: phobias; anxiety disorders • Impulse-control disorders • Obsessive-compulsive personality disorder • Body dysmorphic disorder • Depression • Neurological disorders	• Yale-Brown Obsessive-Compulsive Scale (Y-BOCS) • Psychiatric evaluation; HAM-D, HAM-A • Mental status exam • Neurological exam	• Pharmacological: SSRIs: fluoxetine (higher doses); fluvoxamine; clomipramine • Beta blockers: propranolol • Behavior therapy: exposure and response prevention • Deep muscle relaxation • Individual and family therapy • Education

Trauma- and Stressor-Related Disorders

The disorders within this new classification were originally listed under *Disorders of Infancy, Childhood, and Adolescence; Anxiety Disorders*, and also *Adjustment Disorders* in the DSM-IV-TR (APA 2000).

DSM-5 Trauma and Stressor-Related Disorders

- Acute Stress Disorder
- Adjustment Disorders
- Disinhibited Social Engagement Disorder
- Posttraumatic Stress Disorder
- Reactive Attachment Disorder
- Other Specified or Unspecified Trauma- and Stressor-Related Disorder (APA 2013) (See listing of disorders in *Tools* Tab.)
- *Reactive Attachment Disorder of Infancy or Early Childhood* has been split into two disorders in the DSM-5: *Reactive Attachment Disorder* and *Disinhibited Social Engagement Disorder*. Ongoing systematic research favored two distinct disorders (Zeanah 2010).
- *Acute Stress Disorder* and *Posttraumatic Stress Disorder* moved from the *Adjustment Disorders* and the *Anxiety Disorders* classifications in DSM-IV-TR (APA 2000).

Adjustment Disorders

- Emotional or behavioral reaction to an identifiable stressor within 3 mo of stressor. Marked distress affecting work, social life, and other functional areas; out of proportion to stressor severity.
- Following the death of a loved one, symptoms do not represent normal bereavement.
- Once stressor has ended, symptoms do not continue for more than 6 additional months.
- *Added specifiers*: With depressed mood, with anxiety, with mixed anxiety and depressed mood, and others (APA 2013).

Acute Stress Disorder

- Minor modifications and changes from the DSM-IV-TR (APA 2000).
- Exposure to death, injury, sexual violation; witnessing events; or events involving a close family member or friend. Can result in intrusion

symptoms, dissociative symptoms, avoidance, and arousal symptoms, lasting 3 days to 1 mo. Significant distress in work, social, other areas of functioning (APA 2013).

Reactive Attachment Disorder (RAD)

- RAD was previously listed under the classification *Disorders of Infancy, Childhood, and Adolescence* in the DSM-IV-TR (APA 2000).
- Child is at least 9 mo and less than 5 y demonstrating developmentally inappropriate attachment behaviors and rarely seeks comfort from attachment figures.
- Lacks social/emotional responsiveness, and does not meet autism spectrum disorder (ASD) criteria.
- *Pathogenic care:* Caregivers are neglectful, caregiver disregard for physical needs, repeated changes of caregivers or institutional setting with poor staff ratios. These are believed to be the causes of the attachment disorder (APA 2013).

Disinhibited Social Engagement Disorder

- *New to the DSM-5.*
- Child approaches and interacts with unfamiliar adults, with two of following: reduced reservation about approaching unfamiliar adult, overly familiar and violates social/cultural boundaries, doesn't check back with caregiver, or willing to go with unfamiliar person without reservation.
- Related to the pathogenic care found in RAD and developmental age of at least 9 mo (APA 2013).

Posttraumatic Stress Disorder (PTSD)

- *DSM-5:* Clearer definition of PTSD and excludes PTSD from viewing movies, photos, TV, etc. Must directly experience an event, witness an event, or event experienced by close family member or friend. Now includes *criteria*, such as 1) distorted blame of self or others, 2) persistent negative emotions, and 3) reckless or self-destructive behavior.
- The current three diagnostic clusters of PTSD will be replaced by four clusters consisting of the following criteria: (B) Intrusion Symptoms, (C) Persistent Avoidance, (D) Alterations in Cognitions and Mood, and (E) Hyperarousal and Reactivity Symptoms.
- *Eliminated acute and chronic specifier.* Added subtypes: Preschool (< 9 y) and Dissociative subtypes (APA 2013).
- *Cross-cultural and developmental factors* will be considered.
- See PTSD *Treatments* end of Psychiatric Interventions section, this Tab.

Posttraumatic Stress Disorder (PTSD)

Signs & Symptoms	Causes	Rule Outs	Labs/Tests/Exams	Interventions
• Traumatic event (self/family/witness others); threat of harm or death of actual death and helplessness; does not include viewing movies/TV • Intrusive symptoms • Hyperarousal symptoms • Avoidance symptoms • Persistent anxiety; outbursts (anger/ aggression); negative cognitions/mood; PTSD for children 6 years or younger (APA 2013)	• Rape, torture, child abuse, natural disaster, war, terrorism, etc. • Physiological/ neurochemical/ endocrinological disorder • Sympathetic hyperarousal • Limbic system (amygdala dysfunction) • "Kindling": ↑↓ • Risk factor: previous trauma • Combat military 3-fold increase since 2001 • Lifetime prevalence ~8% (U.S.) (APA 2013)	• Acute stress disorder (clinician-administered) • Obsessive-compulsive disorder • Adjustment disorder • Depression • Panic disorder • Psychotic disorders • Substance-induced disorder • Psychotic disorder due to a general medical condition • Dissociative disorders	• PTSD scale • Primary Care-PTSD Screen (Prins 2003) • Psychiatric evaluation (Shapiro 2001) • Suicidal Behaviors Questionnaire-R • Mental status exam • Neurological exam • CAGE, SMAST • Physical exam, routine blood studies • No laboratory test can diagnose	• Debriefing (rescuers) • Individual or group psychotherapy • CBT/Mindfulness • Eye Movement Desensitization and Reprocessing (EMDR) • Prolonged exposure therapy (See PTSD Treatments this Tab) • Pharmacotherapy: Antidepressants – SSRIs, SNRIs, MAOIs, TCAs; antipsychotics; anxiolytics; mood stabilizers • Family and community support/ art therapy/ psychodrama • PTSD Coach (free mobile app)

Somatic Symptom and Related Disorders

Previously listed as the *Somatoform Disorders* in DSM-IV-TR (APA 2000).

DSM-5 Somatic Symptom Disorders

- Somatic Symptom Disorder
- Illness Anxiety Disorder
- Conversion Disorder (Functional Neurological Symptom Disorder)
- Psychological Factors Affecting Other Medical Conditions
- Factitious Disorder
- Other Specified or Unspecified Somatic Symptom and Related Disorder

(APA 2013) (A full list of disorders in *Tools* Tab.)

Somatic Symptom Disorder

- *Somatic Symptom Disorder* is a new disorder to the DSM-5 taking shared common features from *Somatization Disorder, Undifferentiated Somatoform Disorder, Pain Associated With Both Psychological and General Medical Conditions* and the *Pain Disorders* in the DSM-IV-TR (APA 2000).
- Deemphasizes the role of medical symptoms and emphasizes positive signs and symptoms (distress, excessive thoughts, feelings, and behaviors) (APA 2013).

Illness Anxiety Disorder

- *Illness Anxiety Disorder* replaces *hypochondriasis* and is a milder form of somatic symptom disorder, although it still requires persistence and needs to exist for at least 6 mo. *Fears* serious illness, without symptoms.

Other Somatic Symptom Disorders

- *Factitious Disorder* moved to this classification from its own classification in DSM-IV-TR (APA 2000) to improve research on the disorder. Feigned physical/psychological illness to assume sick role. Unlike malingering, external incentives, including economic gain or avoidance (of responsibility) are absent. *Subtypes:* imposed on self or imposed on another (APA 2013).
- *Conversion Disorder* and *Psychological Factors Affecting Medical Conditions* have minor changes and have been streamlined (APA 2013).

Somatic Symptom Disorder (SSD)

Signs & Symptoms	Causes	Rule Outs	Labs/Tests/Exams	Interventions
• One or more somatic sx: distressing and interfering in daily life • Excessive thoughts, feelings, behaviors about sx: specify severity: mild, moderate, or severe • Disproportionate to seriousness; high anxiety, or ↑ time devoted to sx • Chronic: Persists >6 mo (APA 2013)	• Prevalence rate in general adult population about 5%–7% • Observed in 10%–20% of female first-degree relatives with SD • Females report more somatic symptoms than males; SSD likely higher in females than males (APA 2013)	• General medical condition • Mental status exam (exercise) • Illness anxiety disorder • Panic disorder • Depressive disorder • Anxiety disorder • Conversion disorder • OCD; body dysmorphic disorder	• Psychiatric evaluation • PHQ-12 Somatic Symptom Scale • Neurological exam • Physical exam, routine blood studies • No lab test is remarkable for these subjective complaints • Must R/O medical condition	• Antidepressants • Stress management • Lifestyle changes (exercise) • Collaboration between primary care physician and mental health provider (MHP) • Psychotherapy • CBT • Psychoeducation • Family support • Support/understanding – client often believes sym-ptoms are physical/refuses psychological help • Avoid unnecessary medical treatments/tests (often doctor/hospital shops) • Chronic fluctuating disorder – rarely remits

Sexual Dysfunctions

Previously *Sexual and Gender Identity Disorders* in the DSM-IV-TR (2000), renamed *Sexual Dysfunctions*. *Gender Identity Disorder* renamed *Gender Dysphoria* and given its own classification (DSM-5 [APA 2013]).

In order to understand dysfunction, sexual health needs to be defined and understood.

- *Sexual health* is defined as a state of physical, emotional, mental, and social well-being related to sexuality; it is not merely the absence of disease or dysfunction. It requires a respectful and positive approach, free of coercion, discrimination, and violence. Sexual practices are safe and have the possibility of pleasure (WHO 1975).
- A person's *sex* refers to biological characteristics that define this person as a male or a female (some individuals possess both male and female biological characteristics [hermaphrodite/intersex]) (WHO 2002).
- *Gender* refers to the characteristics of men and women that are socially constructed rather than biologically determined. People are taught the behaviors and roles that result in their becoming men and women, also known as gender identity and gender roles (APA 2000). (See *Gender Dysphoria* in this Tab.)
- *Sexual orientation* refers to the sexual preference of a person, whether male to female, female to male, or bisexual. Variations in sexual preference are considered to be sexually healthy (APA 2000).
- *Sexual dysfunction* is a disturbance in the sexual response cycle or is associated with pain during intercourse.
- *Sexual response cycle dysfunctions* include the areas of desire, excitement, orgasm, and resolution.

DSM-5 Sexual Dysfunction Disorders

- Delayed Ejaculation
- Premature (Early) Ejaculation
- Erectile Disorder
- Female Orgasmic Disorder
- Female Sexual Interest/Arousal Disorder
- Genito-Pelvic Pain/Penetration Disorder
- Male Hypoactive Sexual Desire Disorder
- Substance/Medication-Induced Sexual Dysfunction
- Other Specified or Unspecified Sexual Dysfunction

(See full listing of disorders in *Tools* Tab.) (APA 2013)

Female Sexual Interest/Arousal Disorder

Signs & Symptoms	Causes	Rule Outs	Labs/Tests/Exams	Interventions
• Lack of interest/ arousal ≥6 mo • Absent/reduced frequency/intensity: • Interest • Sexual thoughts • Unreceptive to partner initiating • Sexual excitement • Response to cues • Response to genital sensations • Significant distress experienced (APA 2013)	• Psychological: partner incompatibility, anger, sexual dysphoria issues, sexual preference issues, negative parental views about sex (as a child) • Inhibitions due to cultural/religious influences/beliefs	• Extremes in sexual appetite (sexual addict as a partner) • Major depression • Medical condition • Substance use • Medication • Sexual abuse	• Complete physical exam, including medical history • Psychiatric evaluation • Mental status exam • Sexual history • Routine lab work, thyroid function tests • HAM-D, BDI • SMAST, • CAGE	• Refer to sex therapist • Relationship therapy • CBT • Assuming no physical/medication/ substance use disorder, deal with relationship issues (communication skills) and assure sexual compatibility and sexual orientation

Paraphilic Disorders

- The *Paraphilic Disorders* involve sexually arousing fantasies, urges, or behaviors triggered by/focused on nonhuman objects, self, or partner humiliation, nonconsenting adults, or children, which are recurrent for a period of at least 6 months.
- There are episodic paraphilics that operate only during times of stress.
- Previously included under the *Sexual and Gender Identity Disorders* in the DSM-IV-TR (APA 2000), is now its own classification (APA 2013).

DSM-5 Paraphilic Disorders

- Exhibitionistic Disorder
- Fetishistic Disorder
- Frotteuristic Disorder
- Pedophilic Disorder
- Sexual Masochism Disorder
- Sexual Sadism Disorder
- Transvestic Disorder
- Voyeuristic Disorder
- Other Specified or Unspecified Paraphilic Disorder (APA 2013)

Gender Dysphoria

In the DSM-IV-TR, *Gender Dysphoria* was included with the *Sexual Disorders* (APA 2000) as *Gender Identity Disorder* and now has been renamed and assigned its own classification.

- *Gender* refers to the characteristics of men and women that are *socially constructed* rather than biologically determined. People are taught the *behaviors* and *roles* that result in their becoming men and women, also known as *gender identity* and *gender roles*.
- Gender roles are also culturally determined and differ from one culture to another; they are not static; they are also affected by the law and religious practice.
- Gender also relates to power relationships (between men and women) as well as reproductive rights issues and responsibilities.

DSM-5 Gender Dysphoria Disorders

- Gender Dysphoria in Children
- Gender Dysphoria in Adolescents and Adults (APA 2013)

Gender Identity Disorder (DSM-IV-TR) was transitionally renamed *Gender Incongruence* (as seen as the core issue), but there was concern that "incongruence" could apply to others with gender atypical behaviors. It was finally decided that "dysphoria" best described the significant distress associated with this condition (APA 2013). (See Tools Tab for full list of Disorders.)

Gender Dysphoria

- There is a marked incongruence between experienced gender and assigned gender for at least 6 mo.
- Clinically significant distress or impairment in important functional areas.
- Strong conviction that one is of the other gender.
- Children have a strong desire to play with toys and playmates of other gender (APA 2013).

Sexual Dysfunctions/Paraphilic Disorders/Gender Dysphoria – Client/Family Education

Sexual Dysfunctions

- Clients and their partners need to understand where in the sexual response cycle the problem exists (arousal/orgasm).
- If the problem is one of desire or aversion, this needs to be explored further to determine the causes: couple discord, gender dysphoria, sexual orientation issues, negative views of sexual activity, previous sexual abuse, body image, or self-esteem issues.
- The same holds true for other sexual dysfunctions (orgasmic problems/erectile dysfunction) in that issues around substance use/abuse; previous sexual experiences; possible psychological, physical, and other stressors as factors, including medical conditions and prescribed medications, need to be explored.
- Referral to a sex therapist may be needed to find ways to reconnect intimately. Sometimes partner education is needed on how to satisfy the other partner (mutual satisfaction).

Paraphilic Disorders/Gender Dysphoria

Paraphilic Disorders require help from professionals especially trained in dealing with these disorders. *Gender Dysphoria* also requires psychological professionals who specialize in gender issues, as well as a team of experts (medical) that can manage sex reassignment if/when client takes that step.

- Sexual and other disorders involve cultural considerations, moral and ethical concerns, religious beliefs, and legal considerations. Need to evaluate own beliefs, values, possible prejudices, and comfort level in dealing with these disorders.

Feeding and Eating Disorders

- *Eating disorders* are influenced by many factors, including family rituals and values around food and eating, ethnic and cultural influences, societal influences, and individual biology.
- American society currently stresses physical beauty and fitness and favors the thin and slim female as the ideal.
- There has been a dramatic increase in the number of obese people in the United States – at an alarming rate among children.
- With society's emphasis on fast and convenient foods, high in calories, a reduction in exercise (computers/TV), and the ongoing value of "thin as beautiful," eating disorders remain a concern.

DSM-5 Feeding and Eating Disorders

- Anorexia Nervosa
- Avoidant/Restrictive Food Intake Disorder
- Binge Eating Disorder
- Bulimia Nervosa
- Pica
- Rumination Disorder
- Other Specified or Unspecified Feeding or Eating Disorder

(APA 2013) (See full listing of disorders in *Tools* Tab.)

Pica and Rumination Disorder were previously under *Disorders First Diagnosed in Infancy/Childhood; Avoidant/Restrictive Food Intake Disorder* was formerly *Feeding Disorder of Infancy or Early Childhood* (DSM-IV-TR (APA 2000)). All feeding and eating disorders (infancy, childhood, adolescence, and adulthood) have now been placed within this one classification (Feeding and Eating Disorders) in the DSM-5 (APA 2013).

Anorexia Nervosa/Bulimia Nervosa

- Two common eating disorders are *Anorexia Nervosa* (AN) and *Bulimia Nervosa* (BN). Both use/manipulate eating behaviors in an effort to control weight. Each has its dangers and consequences if maintained over time. (See the table on *Bulimia Nervosa* for signs and symptoms and treatments.) Need to monitor levels of severity.
- *Anorexia Nervosa* – The AN client is terrified of gaining weight and does not maintain a minimally acceptable body weight.

- There is a definite disturbance in the perception of the size or shape of the body.
- AN is more common in industrialized societies and can begin as early as age 13 y.
- Monitor severity based on BMI (mild, moderate, severe, or extreme) to determine disability, treatment.
- Even though underweight, client still fears becoming overweight.
- Self-esteem and self-evaluation based on weight and body shape.
- Amenorrhea develops, as defined by absence of three consecutive menstrual cycles (APA 2013).

Binge Eating Disorder

Previously listed in the *Appendix* of the DSM-IV-TR (APA 2000) *for further study*, but now a *new disorder* in the DSM-5 (APA 2013).

- Eating portions larger than normal, lack of control over eating; also 3 or more: 1) more rapidly, 2) until uncomfortably full, 3) large amounts when not hungry, 4) embarrassed by amounts, or 5) disgusted, depressed, guilty after eating.
- Marked distress over eating; at least once weekly for 3 mo (APA 2013).

Client/Family Education – Eating Disorders

- Client and family need to understand the serious nature of eating disorders; mortality rate for AN clients is 2%–8% (30%–40% recover; 25%–30% improve; 15%–20% do not improve). About 50% of BN clients recover with treatment (Rakel 2000).
- Team approach important – client and family need to be involved with the team, which should or may include a nutritionist, psychiatrist, therapist, physician, psychiatric nurse, nurse, eating disorder specialist, and others.
- Teach client coping strategies, allow for expression of feelings, teach relaxation techniques, and help with ways (other than food) to feel in control.
- Family therapy important to work out parent-child issues, especially around control (should have experience with eating disorders).
- Focus on the fact that clients do recover and improve, and encourage patience when there is a behavioral setback.

Elimination Disorders

Previously included within *Disorders Usually First Diagnosed in Infancy, Childhood, and Adolescence* in the DSM-IV-TR (APA 2000).

- Enuresis or Encopresis (DSM-5; APA 2013)

Bulimia Nervosa (BN)

Signs & Symptoms	Causes	Rule Outs	Labs/Tests/Exams	Interventions
• Recurrent binge eating of large amount of food over short period • Lack of control and cannot stop • Self-induced vomiting, laxatives, fasting, exercise to compensate • At least 1×/wk for 3 mo • Normal weight; some underweight/ overweight • Tooth enamel erosion/ finger or pharynx bruising • Fluid and electrolyte disturbances (APA 2013)	• Genetic predisposition • Hypothalamic dysfunction implication • Family hx of mood disorders and obesity • Issues of power and control • Societal emphasis on thin • Affects 1%–3% women (APA 2013) • Develops late adolescence through adulthood	• Anorexia nervosa • Binge-eating Disorder • Major depressive disorder (MDD) with atypical features • BPD • General medical conditions: Kleine-Levin syndrome • Endocrine disorders	• Complete physical exam • Psychiatric evaluation • Mental status exam • Routine lab work, including TFT, CBC, electrolytes, UA • HAM-D; BDI • MDQ • ECG • SMAST • CAGE	• Individual, group, marital, family therapy • Behavior modification • Nutritional support • Medical support; monitor severity level: mild, moderate, severe, extreme • Client-family education/ support

Personality Disorders

The DSM-5 (APA 2013) has retained all ten personality disorders (PDs) from the DSM-IV-TR (APA 2000), although it proposed eliminating four (*dependent, histrionic, paranoid, and schizoid*) (APA 2012) and instead focusing on often shared common traits among all the disorders.

The APA task force had proposed a hybrid "dimensional" approach to PDs for the DSM-5, rather than limiting to ten specific PDs with discrete criteria. However, it was decided by the APA (Board of Trustees) that a change at this point would be too drastic and could result in diagnostic complexities beyond how clinicians were trained and how they were used to diagnosing PDs (APA 2012).

- The *personality disorders* have been described as an *inflexible* and *maladaptive* way of relating to and perceiving the world.
- It is believed that the *pattern is enduring* and affects all areas of a person's life: occupational, social, and personal.
- The pattern can be traced back to *adolescence* and *early adulthood* and may affect "affect," impulse control, cognition, and interpersonal functioning.
- The "enduring" description is being questioned as many disorders are in fact enduring. It is often believed those with a personality disorder (especially borderline personality disorder) cannot change or be helped. Current treatments and motivation to change can, in fact, result in successes and improved functioning and better relationships.

DSM-5 Personality Disorders

- Cluster A: Paranoid Personality Disorder
- Cluster A: Schizoid Personality Disorder
- Cluster A: Schizotypal Personality Disorder
- Cluster B: Antisocial Personality Disorder
- Cluster B: Borderline Personality Disorder
- Cluster B: Histrionic Personality Disorder
- Cluster B: Narcissistic Personality Disorder
- Cluster C: Avoidant Personality Disorder
- Cluster C: Dependent Personality Disorder
- Cluster C: Obsessive-Compulsive Personality Disorder
- Other Personality Disorders

(APA 2013) (See full listing of disorders in *Tools* Tab.)

Alternative DSM-5 Model for Personality Disorders

- Leaning toward a hybrid "dimensional approach" to the personality disorders, the APA proposed focusing on the general criteria/primary *features of any personality disorder, which are Impairments in Personality Functioning* (self and interpersonal) and *Pathological Trait Domains*.
  - The *Impairments in Personality* were to be evaluated using the *Level of Personality Functioning Scale (LPFS)*, which would measure *Self Functioning* (identity or self-direction) and *Interpersonal Functioning* (empathy or intimacy)
  - If significant impairment existed in *Self and Interpersonal Functioning*, then *Pathological Personality Trait Domains* were to be identified.
- The *Pathological Personality Trait Domains* are higher-order trait domains:
  1. *Negative Affectivity*
  2. *Detachment*
  3. *Antagonism*
  4. *Disinhibition*
  5. *Psychoticism*

The *trait facets*, a more specific and descriptive subset, would then need to be identified to add further dimensions to evaluate and eventually determine treatment. Trait facets included emotional lability, restricted affectivity, manipulativeness, risk taking, and unusual beliefs to name a few (dsm5.org 2012 [DSM-5, Section III, 2013]).

- The APA (2012) has decided that the above proposed changes to the personality disorders should not be implemented during release of this edition of the DSM-5. The **Alternative Model** is listed in Section III of the DSM-5 (Emerging Measures and Models) to allow clinicians time to become familiar with it, but the categorical model remains in Section II of the DSM-5 for clinical use (APA 2013).

Borderline Personality Disorder

Signs & Symptoms	Causes	Rule Outs	Labs/Tests/Exams	Interventions
• Pattern of unstable relationships • Fear of abandonment • Splitting: idealize and devalue (love/hate) • Impulsive: sex, substance abuse, binge eating, reckless driving • Suicidal gestures/self-injury • Intense mood changes lasting a few hours • Chronic emptiness • Intense anger • Transient paranoid ideation (APA, 2013)	• Genetic predisposition • Family hx of mental disorders; may be a variant of/related to bipolar or, MDD • Physical/sexual abuse • About 6% of primary-care population • Predominantly female (75%) (APA, 2013)	• May have comorbid mental disorders, depressive/bipolar • Psychiatric evaluation • Mental status exam • Substance use • General medical condition (due to)	• Millon Clinical Multiaxial Inventory-III (MCMI-II) • Psychiatric evaluation • Mental status exam • HAM-D; BDI • HAM-A; CAGE • SMAST • Physical exam, routine lab work, TFT; monitor self injury	• Linehan (1993) dialectical behavior therapy (DBT) • CBT • Group, individual, family therapy (long-term therapy) • Special strategies • Boundary setting • Be aware that these can be difficult clients even for experienced MH professionals • Pharmacotherapy: antidepressants, mood stabilizers, antipsychotics; caution with benzodiazepines (dependence)

Personality Disorders – Client/Family Education

- Share personality disorder with client and family and educate about the disorder. In this way the client has a basis/framework to understand his/her patterns of behavior.
- Work with client and family in identifying most troublesome behaviors (temper tantrums), and work with client on alternative responses and to anticipate triggers.
- For clients who act out using suicidal gestures, an agreement may have to be prepared that helps client work on impulse control. Agreement might set an amount of time that client will not mutilate and what client will do instead (call a friend/therapist/listen to music). Need to teach alternative behaviors.
- It is better to lead clients to a conclusion ("Can you see why your friend was angry when you did such and such?") rather than tell the client what he or she did to offend person.
- Although BPD receives much attention, all clients with personality disorders (narcissist, antisocial, avoidant personalities) suffer in relationships, occupations, social situations.
- Client needs to be ready and motivated to change, and a therapeutic (trusting) relationship is a prerequisite for anyone with a personality disorder to accept criticisms/frustrations. Some clients believe the problems rest with everyone but themselves.
- Helpful books for BPD clients and families to read in order to understand the borderline personality include: Kreisman JJ, Straus H. I Hate You – Don't Leave Me [rev], Perigee, 2010, and Kreisman JJ, Straus H. Sometimes I Act Crazy: Living with Borderline Personality Disorder, Hoboken, NJ, John Wiley & Sons, 2006.
- For professionals: Linehan MM. Skills Training Manual for Treating Borderline Personality Disorder, New York, Guilford Press, 1993, and Linehan MM. Cognitive-Behavioral Treatment of Borderline Personality Disorder, New York, Guilford Press, 1993.

Neurodevelopmental Disorders

The following disorders were previously listed under Disorders Usually First Diagnosed in Infancy, Childhood, or Adolescence in the DSM-IV-TR (APA 2000).

DSM-5 Neurodevelopmental Disorders

■ Intellectual Disabilities
■ Intellectual Disability (Intellectual Developmental Disorder)

- Global Developmental Delay/Unspecified Intellectual Disability
- Communication Disorders
  - Language Disorder
  - Speech Sound Disorder
  - Social (Pragmatic) Communication Disorder
- Autism Spectrum Disorder
  - Autism Spectrum Disorder
- Attention Deficit/Hyperactivity Disorder
  - Attention Deficit/Hyperactivity Disorder
  - Other Specified or Unspecified Attention Deficit/Hyperactivity Disorder
- Specific Learning Disorder
  - Specific Learning Disorder
- Motor Disorders
  - Developmental Coordination Disorder
  - Stereotypic Movement Disorder
  - Tourette's Disorder
  - Persistent (Chronic) Motor or Vocal Tic Disorder
  - Provisional Tic Disorder
  - Other Specified Tic Disorder
  - Unspecified Tic Disorder
  - Other Neurodevelopmental Disorders
- *Intellectual Disability* (previously Mental Retardation) diagnosis requires a current *intellectual deficit* as well as a deficit in *adaptive functioning* with onset during the developmental period (APA 2013) (See full listing of disorders in *Tools* Tab.)

Intellectual Disability	
50–70 MILD	Able to live independently with some assistance; some social skills; does well in structured environment
35–49 MODERATE	Some independent functioning; needs to be supervised; some unskilled vocational abilities (workshop)
20–34 SEVERE	Total supervision; some basic skills (simple repetitive tasks)
<20 PROFOUND	Total care and supervision; care is constant and continual; little to no speech/no social skills ability

Modified from Townsend 6th ed., 2014, with permission.

Autism Spectrum Disorder

- Previously *Autistic Disorder* in DSM-IV-TR (APA 2000), but is now a new *disorder that includes Autistic Disorder, Childhood Disintegrative Disorder, Asperger's,* and *Pervasive Developmental Disorder, Not Otherwise Specified.* Asperger's no longer exists as a separate disorder.
- DSM-5 views these disorders as part of a spectrum based on clinical presentation and pathological findings.
- ASD is determined by impairments in social interaction and communication as well as *fixed interests* and *repetitive behaviors.*
- *Level of severity* is from mild to severe. There are three levels for both *social communication and restricted interests/repetitive behaviors.* Level 1: requires support; Level 2: requires substantial support; and Level 3: requires very substantial support.

Attention Deficit/Hyperactivity Disorder (ADHD)

- *ADHD* is characterized by a pattern of behavior observed in multiple settings causing social, educational, work difficulties for at least 6 mo (APA 2013). Severity levels include mild, moderate, or severe.

Inattention includes:

- Carelessness and inattention to detail
- Cannot sustain attention and does not appear to be listening
- Does not follow through on instructions and unable to finish tasks, chores, homework
- Difficulty with organization and dislikes activities that require concentration and sustained effort
- Loses things; distracted by extraneous stimuli; forgetful

Hyperactivity-impulsivity includes:

- Fidgeting, moving feet, squirming
- Runs about/climbs excessively
- Leaves seat before excused
- Difficulty playing quietly
- "On the go" and "driven by motor"
- Excessive talking
- Blurts out answers, speaks before thinking
- Problem waiting his/her turn
- Interrupts or intrudes
- Impairment is present before age 12 y, and impairment is present in at least two settings (or more) (DSM-5 [APA 2013]). DSM-IV-TR: Impairment was before age 7 (APA 2000). *Specifiers:* Combined presentation, Predominantly Inattentive Presentation, or Predominantly Hyperactive/ Impulsive (APA 2013).

- Interferes with or reduces function in social, occupational, or academic setting. Symptoms are not caused by another disorder. Prevalence rate, school-aged children: about 5% (APA 2013).
- Many possible causes: genetics; biochemical (possible neurochemical deficits [dopamine, NE]); intrauterine exposure to substances such as alcohol or smoking; exposure to lead, dyes, and additives in food; stressful home environments.
- *Adult ADHD* – Study presented at American Psychiatric Association on the prevalence in the US (Farone 2004); ADHD estimated at 4.1% in adults, ages 18–44, in a given year (NIMH 2010).

Nonpharmacological ADHD Treatments

- Individual/family therapy
- Behavior modification: clear expectations and limits
- Break commands up into clear steps
- Support desired behaviors and immediately respond to undesired behaviors with consequences
- Natural consequences helpful (loses bicycle; do not replace; has to save own money to replace)
- Time-outs may be needed for cooling down/reflecting
- *Role playing*: helpful in teaching friend-friend interactions; helps child prepare for interactions and understand how intrusive behaviors annoy and drive friends away
- *Inform school*: important that school knows about ADHD diagnosis, as this is a disability (Americans with Disabilities Act)
- Seek out special education services
- *Classroom*: sit near teacher, one assignment at a time, written instructions, untimed tests, tutoring (need to work closely with teacher and explain child's condition [ADHD])
- *Nutritional*: many theories remain controversial but include food sensitivities (Feingold diet, allergen elimination, leaky gut syndrome, Nambudripad's allergy elimination technique), supplementation (thiamine), minerals (magnesium, iron), essential fatty acids, amino acids; evaluate for lead poisoning

For *Pharmacological ADHD Treatments, See Drugs/Labs tab.*

Disruptive, Impulse-Control, and Conduct Disorders

These disorders were previously classified under *Disorders Usually First Diagnosed in Infancy, Childhood, or Adolescence* or *Impulse-Control Disorders Not Elsewhere Classified* in the DSM-IV-TR (APA 2000) and are now grouped in this new DSM-5 classification (APA 2013).

DSM-5 Disruptive, Impulse Control, Conduct Disorders

- Conduct Disorder
- Antisocial Personality Disorder
- Intermittent Explosive Disorder
- Oppositional Defiant Disorder
- Pyromania/Kleptomania (APA 2013)

Conduct Disorder/Oppositional Defiant Disorder

- *Conduct disorder (CD)* (serious rule violation, aggression [people/animals], destruction) is a persistent pattern of behavior where the rights of others are violated, and *oppositional defiant disorder (ODD)* (negative, hostile, defiant) is a pattern of irritable, angry mood and argumentative and defiant behaviors (APA 2013).
- *Subtypes for CD* will include childhood onset, adolescent onset, and unspecified onset. Levels of severity: Mild, moderate or severe.
- An *additional specifier* is With Limited Prosocial Emotions in CD.
- *Serious comorbidities* include CD/ADHD, ODD/ADHD, and CD/ADHD/GAD/ MDD. (See full listing of disorders in *Tools Tab*.)

Sleep-Wake Disorders

Previously *Sleep Disorders* in the DSM-IV-TR (APA 2000) and now adds "wake" to the classification, DSM-5 is looking to educate clinicians further about these disorders that have psychological as well as medical/neurological aspects. Some disorders will require objective testing, such as polysomnography and hypocretin measurements for narcolepsy (APA 2013).

DSM-5 Sleep-Wake Disorders

- Central Sleep Apnea
- Circadian Rhythm Sleep-Wake Disorders
- Disorder of Arousal
- Hypersomnolence Disorder
- Insomnia Disorder
- Narcolepsy
- Nightmare Disorder
- Obstructive Sleep Apnea Hypopnea
- Rapid Eye Movement Sleep Behavior Disorder
- Restless Legs Syndrome (new)

- Sleep-Related Hypoventilation
- Substance/Medication-Induced Sleep Disorder

(APA 2013) (See full listing of disorders in *Tools* Tab.)

Dissociative Disorders

Dissociative Fugue previously in the DSM-IV-TR (APA 2000) has been dropped as a disorder in the DSM-5 (now a specifier for Dissociative Amnesia) and *Derealization* added to *Depersonalization Disorder* (APA 2013).

DSM-5 Dissociative Disorders

- Depersonalization-Derealization Disorder
- Dissociative Amnesia (Dissociative Fugue now a specifier)
- Dissociative Identity Disorder
- Other Specified or Unspecified Dissociative Disorder (APA 2013)

Suicidal Behavior Disorder/Nonsuicidal Self-Injury

- *Suicidal Behavior Disorder* and *Nonsuicidal Self-Injury* did not exist in the DSM-IV-TR (APA 2000), and were proposed by the DSM-5 Task Force as new disorders to be included in the DSM-5. The APA (2012) says that there is "misleading information about suicidal behavior and that without a diagnosis, we are unable to institute preventive measures and drug monitoring." However, **neither disorder will be included as a new disorder in the DSM-5 and both have been moved to Section III for further research (APA 2012/2013).**
- *Suicidal behavior* needs to be differentiated from *nonsuicidal self-injury*, which is done to relieve some psychological distress and involves an *urge* and *preoccupation* with self-injury, without intent to commit suicide (dsm5.org 2012).

(See *Suicidal Behaviors Questionnaire-R* in *Assessment* tab)

Disorders for Further Study

Some disorders considered for the DSM-5, but not included, have moved to Section III as *Conditions for Further Study*:

- Caffeine use disorder
- Attenuated psychosis syndrome
- Persistent complex bereavement disorder
- Internet Gaming Disorder
- Suicidal behavior disorder
- Nonsuicidal self-injury

Psychiatric Interventions

Therapeutic Relationship/Alliance

- The *therapeutic relationship* is not concerned with the skills of the mental health professional (MHP) but rather with the attitudes and the relationship between the MHP and the client. This relationship comes out of the creation of a safe environment, conducive to communication and trust.
- An *alliance* is formed when the professional and the client are working together cooperatively in the best interest of the client. The therapeutic relationship begins the moment the MHP and client first meet (Shea 1999).

Core Elements of a Therapeutic Relationship

- Communication/rapport – It is important to establish a connection before a relationship can develop. Encouraging the client to speak, using open-ended questions, is helpful. Asking general (not personal) questions can relax the client in an initial session. It is important to project a caring, nonjudgmental attitude.
- *Trust* – A core element of a therapeutic relationship. Many clients have experienced disappointment and unstable, even abusive, relationships. Trust develops over time and remains part of the process. Without trust, a therapeutic relationship is not possible. Other important elements are confidentiality, setting boundaries, and consistency.
- *Dignity/Respect* – Many clients have been abused and humiliated and have low self-esteem. If treated with dignity through the therapeutic relationship, clients can learn to regain their dignity.
- *Empathy* – Empathy is not sympathy (caught up in client's feelings) but is, rather, open to understanding the "client's perceptions" and helps the client understand these better through therapeutic exploration.
- *Genuineness* – Genuineness relates to trust because it says to the client: I am honest, and I am a real person. Again, it will allow the client to get in touch with her/his "real" feelings and to learn from and grow from the relationship.

Therapeutic Use of Self

Ability to use one's own personality consciously and in full awareness to establish relatedness and to structure interventions (Travelbee 1971). Requires self-awareness and self-understanding.

Phases of Relationship Development

- *Orientation phase* – This is the phase when the MHP and client first meet and initial impressions are formed.
- Rapport is established, and trust begins.
- The relationship and the connection are most important.
- Client is encouraged to identify the problem(s) and become a collaborative partner in helping self.
- Once rapport and a connection are established, the relationship is ready for the next phase.
- *Identification phase* – In this phase the MHP and client are:
  - Clarifying perceptions and setting expectations in and for the relationship.
  - Getting to know and understand each other.
- *Exploitation (working) phase* – The client is committed to the process and to the relationship and is involved in own self-help; takes responsibility and shows some independence.
  - This is known as the *working phase* because this is when the hard work begins.
  - Client must believe and know that the MHP is caring and *on his/her side* when dealing with the more difficult issues during therapeutic exploration.
  - *It this phase is entered too early,* before trust is developed, clients may suddenly terminate if presented with painful information.
- *Resolution phase* – The client has gained all that he/she needs from the relationship and is ready to leave.
  - This may involve having met stated goals or resolution of a crisis.
  - Be aware of fear of abandonment and need for closure.
  - Both the MHP and client may experience sadness, which is normal.
  - Dependent personalities may need help with termination, reflecting upon the positives and the growth that has taken place through the relationship (Peplau 1992).
- If a situation brings a client back for therapy, the relationship has already been established (trust); therefore, *there is not a return to the orientation phase.* Both will identify new issues and re-establish expectations of proposed outcomes. It will now be *easier to move into the working phase of the relationship,* and this will be done more quickly.

CLINICAL PEARL: Trust and safety are core elements of a therapeutic alliance, as many clients have experienced abuse, inconsistency, broken promises, and "walking on eggs."

Nonverbal Communication

Nonverbal communication may be a better indication of what is going on with a client than verbal explanations.

- Although verbal communication is important, it is only one component of an evaluation.
- Equally important to develop your skills of observation.
- Some clients are not in touch with their feelings, and only their behaviors (clenched fist, head down, arms crossed) will offer clues to feelings.
- Nonverbal communication may offer the client clues as to how the MHP is feeling as well.
- *Physical appearance* – A neat appearance is suggestive of someone who cares for him/herself and feels positive about self. Clients with schizophrenia or depression may appear disheveled and unkempt.
- *Body movement/posture* – Slow or rapid movements can suggest depression or mania; a slumped posture, depression. Medication-induced body movements and postures include: pseudoparkinsonism (antipsychotic); akathisia (restlessness/moving legs [antipsychotic]). Warmth (smiling) and coldness (crossed arms) are also nonverbally communicated.
- *Touch* – Touch forms a bridge or connection to another. Touch has different meanings based on culture, and some cultures touch more than others. Touch can have a very positive effect, but touching requires permission to do so. Many psychiatric clients have had "boundary violations," so an innocent touch may be misinterpreted.
- *Eyes* – The ability to maintain eye contact during conversation offers clues as to social skills and self-esteem. Without eye contact, there is a "break in the connection" between two people. A lack of eye contact can suggest suspiciousness, something to hide. Remember cultural interpretations of eye contact (see *Assessment tab: Culturally Mediated Beliefs and Practices*).
- *Voice* – Voice can be a clue to the mood of a client. Pitch, loudness, and rate of speech are important clues. *Manic clients* speak loudly, rapidly, and with pressured speech. *Anxious clients* may speak with a high pitch and rapidly. *Depressed clients* speak slowly, and obtaining information may feel like "pulling teeth."

Communication Techniques

Technique	Rationale	Example
Reflecting	Reflects back to clients their emotions, using their own words	Client (C): *John never helps with the housework.* Mental Health Professional (MHP): *You're angry that John doesn't help.*
Silence	Allows client to explore all thoughts/feelings; prevents cutting conversation at a critical point or missing something important	MHP nods with some vocal cues from time to time so C knows MHP is listening but does not interject.
Paraphrasing	Restating, using different words to ensure you have understood the client; helps clarify	C: *My grandkids are coming over today and I don't feel well.* MHP: *Your grandkids are coming over, but you wish they weren't, because you are not well. Is that what you are saying?*
Making observations	Helps client recognize feelings he/she may not be aware of and connect with behaviors	MHP: *Every time we talk about your father you become very sad.*
Open-ended/ broad questions	Encourages client to take responsibility for direction of session; avoids yes/no responses	MHP: *What would you like to deal with in this session?*
Encouragement	Encourages client to continue	MHP: *Tell me more . . . uh huh . . . and then?*
Reframing	Presenting same information from another perspective (more positive)	C: *I lost my keys, couldn't find the report, and barely made it in time to turn my report in.* MHP: *In spite of all that, you did turn your report in.*

Continued

Communication Techniques—cont'd

Technique	Rationale	Example
Challenging idea/belief system	Break through denial or fixed belief; always done with a question	MHP: *Who told you that you were incompetent? Where did you get the idea that you can't say no?*
Recognizing change/recognition	Reinforces interest in client and positive reinforcement (this is not a compliment)	MHP: *I noticed that you were able to start our session today rather than just sit there.*
Clarification	Assures that MHP did not misunderstand; encourages further exploration	MHP: *This is what I thought you said . . .; is that correct?*
Exploring in detail	If it appears a particular topic is important, then the MHP asks for more detail; MHP takes the lead from the client (client may resist exploring further)	MHP: *This is the first time I've heard you talk about your sister; would you like to tell me more about her?*
Focusing	Use when a client is covering multiple topics rapidly (bipolar/anxious) and needs help focusing	MHP: *A lot is going on, but let's discuss the issue of your job loss, as I would like to hear more about that.*
Metaphors/symbols	Sometimes clients speak in symbolic ways and need translation	C: *The sky is just so gray today and night comes so early now.* MHP: *Sounds like you are feeling somber.*
Acceptance	Positive regard and open to communication	MHP: *I hear what you are saying. Yes, uh-huh.* (full attention).

Therapeutic Milieu

- In the therapeutic milieu (*milieu* is French for surroundings or environment), the entire environment of the hospital is set up so that every action, function, and encounter is therapeutic.
- The therapeutic community is a smaller representation of the larger community/society outside.
- The coping skills and learned behaviors within the community will also translate to the larger outside community.

Seven Basic Assumptions:

1. The health in each individual is to be realized and encouraged to grow.
2. Every interaction is an opportunity for therapeutic intervention.
3. The client owns his or her own environment.
4. Each client owns his or her own behavior.
5. Peer pressure is a useful and powerful tool.
6. Inappropriate behaviors are dealt with as they occur.
7. Restrictions and punishment are to be avoided (Skinner 1979).

- Therapeutic milieu difficult to implement in era of managed care (short stays).

Group Therapy/Interventions

Stages of Group Development

I. Initial Stage (In/Out)

- Leader orients the group and sets the ground rules, including confidentiality.
- There may be confusion and questions about the purpose of the group.
- Members question themselves in relation to others and how they will fit in the group.

II. Conflict Stage (Top/Bottom)

- Group is concerned with pecking order, role, and place in group.
- There can be criticism and judgment.
- Therapist may be criticized as group finds its way.

III. Cohesiveness (Working) Stage (Near/Far)

- After conflict comes a group spirit, and a bond and trust develop among the members.
- Concern is now with closeness, and an "us versus them" attitude develops: those in the group versus those *outside the group*.
- Eventually becomes a mature working group.

IV. Termination

- Difficult for long-term groups; discuss well before termination.
- There will be grieving and loss (Yalom 2005).

Leadership Styles

- **Autocratic** – The autocratic leader essentially "rules the roost." He or she is the most important person of the team and has very strong opinions of how and when things should be done. Members of a group are not allowed to make independent decisions, as the autocrat trusts only his/her opinions. The autocrat is concerned with power and control and is very good at persuasion. High productivity/low morale.
- **Democratic** – The democratic leader focuses on the group and empowers the group to take responsibility and make decisions. Problem solving and taking action are important, along with offering alternative solutions to problems (by group members). Lower productivity/high morale.
- **Laissez-Faire** – This leadership style results in confusion because of the lack of direction and noninvolvement; it also results in low productivity and morale (Lippitt & White 1958).

Individual Roles/Difficult Group Members

- **Monopolizer** – Involved in some way in every conversation, offering extensive detail or always presents with a "crisis of the week" (minimizing anyone else's concerns/issues).
  - Has always experienced a similar situation: I know what you mean; my dog died several years ago, and it was so painful I am still not over it.
  - Will eventually cause anger and resentment in the group if leader does not control the situation; dropouts result.
- **Help-rejecting complainer** – Requests help from the group and then rejects each and every possible solution so as to demonstrate the hopelessness of the situation.
  - No one else's situation is as bad as that of the help-rejecting complainer. (You think you have it bad; wait until you hear my story!)
  - Often looks to the group leader for advice and help and competes with others for this help, and because he/she is not happy, no one else can be happy either.
- **Silent client** – Does not participate but observes.
  - Could be fear of self-disclosure, exposing weaknesses. Possibly feels unsafe in leaderless group.
  - Does not respond well to pressure or being put on the spot, but must somehow be respectfully included and addressed.
  - The long-term silent client does not benefit from being in a group, nor does the group, and should possibly withdraw from the group.
- **Boring client** – No spontaneity, no fun, no opinions, and a need to present to the world what the client believes the world wants to see and hear.
  - If you are bored by the client, likely the client is boring.
  - Requires the gradual removal of barriers that have kept the individual buried inside for years.

124

■ Often tolerated by others but seldom missed if leaves the group.
■ **Narcissist** – Lack of awareness of others in the group; seeing others as mere appendages and existing for one's own end; feels special and not part of the group (masses).
   ■ Expects from others but gives nothing.
   ■ Can gain from some groups and leaders.
■ **Psychotic client** – Should not be included in early formative stages of a group.
   ■ If a client who is a member of an established group decompensates, then the group can be supportive because of an earlier connection and knowledge of the nonpsychotic state of the person.
■ **BPD client** – Can be challenging in a group because of emotional volatility, unstable interpersonal relationships, fears of abandonment, anger control issues, to name a few.
   ■ Borderline clients idealize or devalue (splitting) – the leader is at first great and then awful.
   ■ Some borderline group members who connect with a group may be helped as trust develops and borderline client is able to accept some frustrations and mild criticisms (Yalom 2005).

CLINICAL PEARL: It is important to understand that *subgroups* (splitting off or smaller group/unit) can and do develop within the larger group. Loyalty transferred to a subgroup undermines overall goals of larger group (some clients are in and some out). May be indirect hostility to leader. Some subgroups and extragroup activities are positive as long as there is not a splintering from/hostility toward larger group. Group needs to address openly feelings about subgroups and outside activities – if splintering or secretiveness continues, will be a detriment to group's cohesiveness and therapeutic benefit.

Yalom's Therapeutic Factors

The factors involved in and derived from the group experience that help and are of value to group members and therapeutic success are:

■ *Instillation of hope* – Hope that this group experience will be therapeutic and effective.
■ *Universality* – Despite individual uniqueness, there are common denominators that allow for a connection and reduce feelings of being alone in one's plight.
■ *Didactic interaction* – In some instances, instruction and education can help people understand their circumstances, and such information relieves anxiety and offers power, such as understanding cancer, bipolar disorder, or HIV.
■ *Direct advice* – In some groups, advice giving can be helpful when one has more experience and can truly help another (cancer survivor helping newly diagnosed cancer patient). Too much advice giving can impede. Advice giving/talking/refusing tells much about the group members and stage of group.

- *Altruism* – Although altruism suggests a concern for others that is unselfish, it is learning that through giving to others, one truly receives. One can find meaning through giving.
- *Corrective recapitulation of the primary family group* – Many clients develop dysfunctions related to the primary group – *the family of origin*. There are often unresolved relationships, strong emotions, and unfinished business. The group often serves as an opportunity to work out some of these issues as leaders and group members remind each other of primary family members, even if not consciously.
- *Socializing techniques* – Direct or indirect learning of social skills. Helpful to those whose interpersonal relationships have fallen short because of poor social skills. Often provided by group feedback, such as *You always turn your body away from me when I talk and you seem bored.* In many instances, individuals are *unaware* of the behaviors that are disconcerting or annoying to others.
- *Imitative behavior* – Members may model other group members, which may help in exploring new behaviors.

Family Therapy

Family Therapy Models/Theories

- *Intergenerational* – The theory of Murray Bowen (1994) that states problems are multigenerational and pass down from generation to generation until addressed. Requires direct discussion and clarification with previous generation members if possible. Concerned with level of individual differentiation and anxiety, triangles, nuclear family emotional system, and multigenerational emotional process. Therapist must remain a neutral third party.
- *Contextual* – The therapy of Boszormenyi-Nagy that focuses on give and take between family members, entitlement and fulfillment, fairness, and the family ledger (an accounting of debts and merits).
- *Structural* – Developed by Salvador Minuchin and views the family as a social organization with a structure and distinct patterns. Therapist takes an active role and challenges the existing order.
- *Strategic* – Associated with Jay Haley and focuses on problem definition and resolution, using active intervention.
- *Communications* – Focuses on the family and communications in the family and emphasizes reciprocal affection and love; the Satir model.
- *Systemic* – Involves multidimensional thinking and use of paradox (tactics that appear opposite to therapy goals but designed to achieve goals); also called the Milan model.

CLINICAL PEARL: In dealing with families, it is important to have an understanding of how families operate, whatever model is used. A model offers a framework for viewing the family. A family is a subsystem within a larger system (community/society) and will reflect the values and culture of that society. Unlike working with individuals, it is the *family that is the client*.

Genogram

A genogram is a visual diagram of a family over two or three generations. It provides an overview of the family and any significant emotional and medical issues and discord among members. It offers insight into patterns and unresolved issues/conflicts throughout the generations.

Common Genogram Symbols

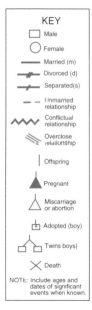

KEY

☐ Male

○ Female

—— Married (m)

Divorced (d)

Separated(s)

- - - Unmarried relationship

Conflictual relationship

Overclose relationship

| Offspring

▲ Pregnant

△ Miscarriage or abortion

Adopted (boy)

Twins boys)

✕ Death

NOTE: Include ages and dates of significant events when known.

■ Other behavioral interventions are: social skills training, assertiveness training, deep-muscle relaxation, exposure and systematic

Sample Genogram

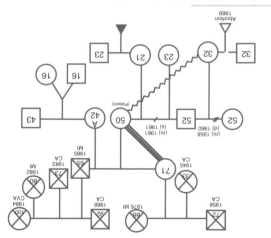

From Townsend 6th ed., 2014, with permission.

Cognitive Behavioral Therapy

■ Cognitive behavioral therapy (CBT) deals with the relationship between cognition, emotion, and behavior.
■ Cognitive aspects are: automatic thoughts, assumptions, and distortions.
■ Individuals are often unaware of the *automatic thoughts* that may affect beliefs and behaviors, such as *I never do well in school* or *I am stupid*.
■ Deep-seated beliefs, or *schemas*, affect perceptions of the world.
■ Individuals are also influenced by *distortions* in their thinking.
■ Important aspects of CBT include agenda setting, review, feedback, and homework.
■ Some techniques may involve treating the behaviors rather than the cognitive aspects.
■ Fearful, dysfunctional clients respond better to behavioral versus cognitive interventions. This may involve task or activity assignments.

desensitization techniques, and in vivo interventions (phobias/agoraphobia) (Freeman et al 2004).

Distortions in Thinking

■ *Catastrophizing* – an uncomfortable event is turned into a catastrophe.
■ *Dichotomous thinking* – either/or thinking, such as I am good or I am evil.
■ *Mind reading* – believes that the person knows what the other is thinking without clarifying.
■ *Selective abstraction* – focusing on one aspect rather than all aspects. Individual hears only the one negative comment during a critique and does not hear the five positive comments.
■ *Fortune telling* – anticipates a negative future event without facts or outcome. *I know I am going to fail that test.*
■ *Overgeneralization* – one event is now representative of the entire situation. A forgotten anniversary is interpreted as the marriage is over and will never be the same.

Mindfulness-Based Cognitive Therapy (MBCT)

MBCT is proving effective in the treatment of recurrent MDD. Mindfulness is an open, accepting, nonjudgmental awareness of self "in the present" and has proved very effective when combined with CBT (Segal 2010).

CLINICAL PEARL: CBT has been shown to be quite effective in treating depression and anxiety disorders (panic/phobia/OCD) and is very helpful when used in conjunction with medication. Through CBT, clients learn to change their thinking and to "reframe" their views/thoughts as well as learn tools/techniques to deal with future episodes. CBT provides the client with a sense of control over his/her fears, depression, and anxiety, as there is an active participation in treatment and outcome. Mindfulness CBT is proving even more effective in some instances, especially depression (Segal 2010).

Treatments for Depression – Nonpharmacological

■ Nonpharmacological treatments are emerging in the treatment of depression, some showing clinical benefit and some needing further study.
  ■ **Vagal nerve stimulation** – uses a small implantable device and is indicated for the adjunctive long-term treatment of chronic or recurrent depression for patients 18 years of age or older who are experiencing a major depressive episode and have not had an adequate response to four or more adequate antidepressant treatments (Cyberonics Inc. 2007; Nemeroff et al 2006).
  ■ **Transcranial magnetic stimulation** – noninvasive, relatively painless novel technique to alter brain physiology (Rachid & Bertschy 2006). More recent study has shown statistically significant and meaningful

antidepressant effect especially in treatment-resistant depression (George 2010).

Integrative Therapies

- *Art therapy* – the use of art media, images, and the creative process to reflect human personality, interests, concerns, and conflicts. Very helpful with children and traumatic memories.
- *Biofeedback* – learned control of the body's physiological responses either voluntarily (muscles) or involuntarily (autonomic nervous system), such as the control of blood pressure or heart rate.
- *Dance therapy* – as the mind/body is connected, dance therapy focuses on direct expression of emotion through the body, affecting feelings, thoughts, and the physical and behavioral responses.
- *Guided imagery* – imagination is used to visualize improved health; has positive effect on physiological responses.
- *Meditation* – self-directed relaxation of body and mind; health-producing benefits through stress reduction.
- *Others:* exercise, humor therapy, deep-muscle relaxation, prayer, acupressure, Rolfing, pet therapy, massage therapy, etc.

CLINICAL PEARL: Never underestimate the benefit of *Integrative Therapies*. In some ways, alternative is a misnomer because these are not alternatives but should be complements to traditional treatments and integrated into the treatment protocols. Both go hand in hand in a comprehensive approach to healing and treatment of the body, mind, and spiritual self. Exercise has been shown to greatly improve depressive symptoms in conjunction with antidepressants (vs. antidepressants alone).

PTSD Treatments

Eye Movement Desensitization and Reprocessing (EMDR)

Developed by Francine Shapiro and involves therapist-directed rapid eye movements that are simultaneously associated with distressing or traumatic thoughts/memories. Bilateral brain stimulation (when eyes are rapidly moved from side to side) helps "reprocess" memories to relieve distress. This has been shown to be an effective treatment for PTSD (Shapiro 2001).

Other PTSD Treatments

Pharmacological interventions, cognitive behavioral therapy, mindfulness CBT, individual and group therapy, and family and community support. Important to begin treatment as soon as possible after diagnosis because of changes in brain physiology and sympathetic activation that become more difficult to treat over time. The Department of Veterans Affairs (http://ptsd.va.gov/) has helpful information and help for soldiers who suffer from PTSD and their families and connects them with other soldiers/families and posts the latest treatments.

Prolonged Exposure Therapy

Prolonged Exposure Therapy is an effective treatment for PTSD that involves *education, breathing, real world practice,* and *talking through the trauma*. It usually involves 8–15, 90-minute sessions (National Center for PTSD 2012).

PTSD Mobile Apps

PTSD Coach – A free educational, self-assessment, and symptom management app for download to a mobile phone for veterans and others with PTSD, though military oriented (Department of Veterans Affairs 2012; http://ptsd.va.gov/).
PE Coach – A free downloadable app to be used during Prolonged Exposure Therapy with a mental health professional (National Center for PTSD 2012).
(See PTSD this Tab; also Terrorism/Disasters as well as Military, Families, and PTSD in Crisis Tab).

Recovery Model

- Mental illness has often been viewed as chronic and debilitating, without expectation of recovery. But in fact recovery is possible for many individuals.
- The *concept of recovery* began in the addictions field and is now being adopted by many professionals in the mental health field. There are many models of recovery (e.g., the Psychological Model of recovery, Tidal Model, etc.).
- In December 2011, SAMHSA announced a working definition of recovery as follows: "A process of change through which individuals improve their health and wellness, live a self-directed life, and strive to reach their full potential."
- SAMHSA also delineated *4 major dimensions* to support recovery: health, home, purpose, and community.
- All models provide guiding principles or steps toward recovery. Information regarding SAMHSA recovery can be found at: http://www.samhsa.gov/recovery/.

Psychotropic Drugs

Labs/Plasma Levels

Psychotropic Drugs

Therapeutic Drug Classes

Antianxiety (Anxiolytic) Agents
Used in the treatment of generalized anxiety, obsessive-compulsive disorder (OCD), posttraumatic stress disorder (PTSD), phobic disorders, insomnia, and others, and include:

- Benzodiazepines (alprazolam, clonazepam, lorazepam, oxazepam)
- Azaspirone (buspirone)
- Alpha-2 adrenergics (clonidine)
- Antihistamines (hydroxyzine)
- Beta blockers (propranolol)
- Antidepressants (doxepin, escitalopram)
- Hypnosedatives for insomnia, such as barbiturates (phenobarbital) and imidazopyridine (zolpidem)

Antidepressant Agents

Used in the treatment of depression, bipolar (depressed), OCD, and others, and include:

- Tricyclics (amitriptyline, desipramine, doxepin, imipramine)
- Monoamine oxidase inhibitors (MAOIs) (phenelzine, tranylcypromine)
- Selective serotonin reuptake inhibitors (SSRIs) (fluoxetine, paroxetine, sertraline)
- Serotonin norepinephrine reuptake inhibitors (SNRIs) (venlafaxine, duloxetine)
- Others (aminoketone/triazolopyridine) (bupropion [Wellbutrin], trazodone [Desyrel]); benzofurans (vilazodone [Viibryd]).

Mood-Stabilizing Agents

Used in the treatment of bipolar disorder (mania/depression), aggression, schizoaffective, and others, and include:

- Lithium
- Anticonvulsants (valproic acid, carbamazepine, lamotrigine, topiramate)
- Calcium channel blockers (verapamil)
- Alpha-2 adrenergics (clonidine) and beta adrenergics (propranolol)

Antipsychotic (Neuroleptic) Agents

Used in the treatment of schizophrenia, psychotic episodes (depression/organic [dementia]/substance-induced), bipolar disorder, agitation, delusional disorder, and others, and include:

- Conventional antipsychotics:
  - phenothiazines (chlorpromazine, thioridazine)
  - butyrophenones (haloperidol)
  - thioxanthenes (thiothixene)
  - diphenylbutyl piperidines (pimozide)

- dibenzoxazepine (loxapine)
- dihydroindolone (molindone)
■ Atypical antipsychotics:
  - dibenzodiazepine (clozapine)
  - benzisoxazole (risperidone)
  - thienobenzodiazepine (olanzapine)
  - benzothiazolyl piperazine (ziprasidone)
  - dihydrocarbostyril (aripiprazole)
  - dibenzo-oxepino pyrroles (asenapine)
  - piperidinyl-benzisoxazole (iloperidone)

(Modified from Pedersen: Pocket Psych Drugs 2010)

Although other agents (e.g., stimulants) may be used in the treatment of psychiatric disorders, the most common therapeutic classes and agents are listed above.

Pharmacokinetics

■ *The Cytochrome P-450 Enzyme System* is involved in drug biotransformation and metabolism. It is important to develop a knowledge of this system to understand drug metabolism and especially drug interactions. Over 30 P-450 isoenzymes have been identified. The major isoenzymes include CYP1A2/2A6/2B6/2C8/2C9/2C18/2C19/2D6/2E1/3A4/3A5-7.

Half-Life is the time (hours) that it takes for 50% of a drug to be eliminated from the body. Time to total elimination involves halving the remaining 50%, and so forth, until total elimination. Half-life is considered in determining dosing frequency and time to steady state. The rule of thumb for **steady state** (stable concentration/manufacture effect) **attainment** is 4–5 half-lives. *Because of fluoxetine's long half-life, a 5-week washout is recommended after stopping fluoxetine and before starting an MAOI to avoid a serious and possibly fatal reaction.*

Protein Binding is the amount of drug that binds to the blood's plasma proteins; the remainder circulates unbound. It is important to understand this concept when prescribing two or more highly protein-bound drugs as one drug may be displaced, causing increased blood levels and adverse effects.

Antipsychotics and Treatment-Emergent Diabetes

Clients receiving atypical antipsychotics (especially clozapine and olanzapine) and also some conventional antipsychotics are at risk for developing diabetes and metabolic syndrome. Many atypicals are being prescribed for adjunctive treatment of depression as well as bipolar disorder. It is critical to monitor weight, BMI, FBS, as well as waist circumference in an effort to anticipate, prevent, and manage these possibilities (Nielsen 2010).

Body Mass Index (BMI)

The intersection of your weight and height equals your BMI. A BMI greater than 30 puts clients at greatest risk for cardiovascular disease/diabetes and other disorders. The preferred BMI is between 19 and 24. Risk increases between 25 and 29 (National Institutes of Health: Clinical Guidelines on the Identification, Evaluation, and Treatment of Overweight and Obesity in Adults: The Evidence Report, September 1998).

Metabolic Syndrome

Metabolic syndrome is defined as a group of clinical symptoms/criteria including abdominal obesity, hypertension, and diabetes, as well as low HDL (high density lipoprotein) levels and high levels of triglycerides. There is now a greater concern about the development of metabolic syndrome for those prescribed antipsychotics (Remington 2006). It is important to monitor waist circumference, BMI, weight, blood pressure, lipids, fasting blood sugar, and Hgb A1C, if diabetic.

Waist circumference should be <40 inches (102 cm) for men and <35 inches (88 cm) for women.

Clinical Identification of the Metabolic Syndrome
Any three of the following:

Risk Factor	Defining Level
Abdominal obesity Men Women	Waist circumference >102 cm (>40 in) >88 cm (>35 in)
Triglycerides	>150 mg/dL
HDL cholesterol Men Women	 <40 mg/dL <50 mg/dL
Blood pressure	>130/>85 mmHg
Fasting glucose	>110 mg/dL

Source: National Institutes of Health. ATP III Guidelines, National Cholesterol Education Program, NIH Publication No. 01-3305.
From Pedersen: Pocket Psych Drugs 2010, with permission.

Attention Deficit Hyperactivity Disorder (ADHD) Agents

Chemical Class	Generic/Trade	Dosage Range/Day
Amphetamines	Dextroamphetamine sulfate (Dexdrine, Dextrostat)	2.5–40 mg
	Methamphetamine (Desoxyn)	5–25 mg
	Lisdexamfetamine (Vyvanse)	20–70 mg
Amphetamine mixtures	Dextroamphetamine/ amphetamine (Adderall, Adderall XR)	2.5–40 mg
Miscellaneous	Methylphenidate (Ritalin; Methylin; Concerta; Metadate; Quillivant XR)	10–60 mg
	Dexmethylphenidate (Focalin)	5–20 mg
	Atomoxetine (Strattera)	>70 kg: 40–100 mg; ≤70 kg: 0.5–1.4 mg/kg (or 100 mg, whichever is less)
	Bupropion (Wellbutrin)	3 mg/kg

From Townsend 2014; Pedersen 2010. Used with permission.

Antiparkinsonian Agents

These are *anticholinergics* used to treat drug-induced parkinsonism, Parkinson's disease, and extrapyramidal symptoms (EPS). These include:

■ Benztropine (Cogentin)
■ Biperiden (Akineton)
■ Trihexyphenidyl (Artane)
■ Amantadine (dopaminergic) and diphenhydramine (antihistaminic) and others

Anticholinergic side effects include:

■ Blurred vision, dry mouth, constipation
■ Sedation, urinary retention, tachycardia

 ⃠ **ALERT:** Use cautiously in the elderly and in cardiac arrhythmias.

Antipsychotic Use Contraindications

- Addison's disease
- Bone marrow depression
- Glaucoma (narrow angle)
- Myasthenia gravis

Antipsychotic-Induced Movement Disorders

Extrapyramidal Symptoms (EPS)

EPS are caused by antipsychotic treatment and need to be monitored/evaluated for early intervention.

- Akinesia – rigidity and bradykinesia
- Akathisia – restlessness; movement of body; unable to keep still; movement of feet (do not confuse with anxiety)
- Dystonia – spasmodic and painful spasm of muscle (torticollis [head pulled to one side])
- Oculogyric crisis – eyes roll back toward the head. This is an emergency situation.
- Pseudoparkinsonism – simulates Parkinson's disease with shuffling gait, drooling, muscular rigidity, and tremor
- Rabbit syndrome – rapid movement of the lips that simulate a rabbit's mouth movements

Tardive Dyskinesia

Permanent dysfunction of voluntary muscles. Affects the mouth – tongue protrudes, smacking of lips, mouth movements,

⊘ **ALERT:** Evaluate clients on antipsychotics for possible tardive dyskinesia by using the Abnormal Involuntary Movement Scale (AIMS) (see AIMS form in Assessment Tab).

Drug-Herbal Interactions

Antidepressants should not be used concurrently with: St. John's wort or SAMe (serotonin syndrome and/or altered antidepressant metabolism).

Benzodiazepines/sedative/hypnotics should not be used concurrently with chamomile, skullcap, valerian, or kava (caution: associated with liver disease and need to check legality by state and country). St. John's wort may reduce the effectiveness of benzodiazepines metabolized by P450 CYP3A4.

Conventional antipsychotics (haloperidol, chlorpromazine) that are sedating should not be used in conjunction with chamomile, skullcap, valerian, or kava.

Carbamazepine, clozapine, and olanzapine should not be used concurrently with St. John's wort (altered drug metabolism/effectiveness).

🚫 **ALERT:** Ask all clients specifically what, if any, herbal or OTC medications they are using to treat symptoms.

Elderly and Medications (Start Low, Go Slow)

- Relevant drug guides provide data about dosing for the elderly and debilitated clients; also see the Geriatric tab as well as Geriatric and Dose Considerations in the Drugs A-Z Tab.
- Elderly or debilitated clients are started at lower doses, often half the recommended adult dose. This is due to:
  - Decreases in GI absorption
  - Decrease in total body water (decreased plasma volume)
  - Decreased lean muscle and increased adipose tissue
  - Reduced first-pass effect in the liver and cardiac output
  - Decreased serum albumin
  - Decreased glomerular filtration and renal tubular secretion
  - Time to steady state is prolonged

Because of decrease in lean muscle mass and increase in fat (retains lipophilic drugs [fat-storing], reduced first-pass metabolism, and decreased renal function, drugs may remain in the body longer and produce an additive effect.

🚫 **ALERT:** With the elderly, start doses low and titrate slowly. Drugs that result in postural hypotension, confusion, or sedation should be used cautiously or not at all.

- **Poor Drug Choices for the Elderly** – Drugs that cause postural hypotension or anticholinergic side effects (sedation).
  - *TCAs* – anticholinergic (confusion, constipation, visual blurring); cardiac (conduction delay; tachycardia); alpha-1 adrenergic (orthostatic hypotension [falls])
  - *Benzodiazepines* – the longer the half-life, the greater the risk of falls. Choose a shorter half-life. Lorazepam (T$\frac{1}{2}$ 12–15 h) is a better choice than diazepam (T$\frac{1}{2}$ 20–70 h; metabolites up to 200 h).
  - *Lithium* – use cautiously in elderly, especially if debilitated.
  - Consider age, weight, mental state, and medical disorders and compare with side-effect profile in selecting medications.

MAOI Diet (Tyramine) Restrictions

Foods: Must Avoid Completely
- Aged red wines (cabernet sauvignon/merlot/chianti)
- Aged (smoked, aged, pickled, fermented, marinated, and processed) meats (pepperoni/bologna/salami, pickled herring, liver, frankfurters, bacon, ham)
- Aged/mature cheeses (blue/cheddar/provolone/brie/Romano/Parmesan/Swiss)
- Overripe fruits and vegetables (overripe bananas/sauerkraut/all overripe fruit)
- Beans (fava, Italian, Chinese pea pod, fermented bean curd, soya sauce, tofu, miso soup)
- Condiments (bouillon cubes/meat tenderizers/canned soups/gravy/sauces/soy sauce)
- Soups (prepared/canned/frozen)
- Beverages (beer/ales/vermouth/whiskey/liqueurs/nonalcoholic wines and beers)

Foods: Use With Caution (Moderation)
- Avocados (not overripe)
- Raspberries (small amounts)
- Chocolate (small amount)
- Caffeine (two, 8-oz. servings per day or less)
- Dairy products (limit to buttermilk, yogurt, and sour cream [small amounts]); cream cheese, cottage cheese, milk OK if fresh

Medications: Must Avoid
- Stimulants
- Decongestants
- OTC medications (check with PCP/pharmacist)
- Opioids
- Meperidine
- Ephedrine/epinephrine
- Methyldopa
- Herbal remedies

Any questions about foods, OTC medications, herbals, medications (newly prescribed) should be discussed with the psychiatrist, pharmacist, or advanced practice nurse because of serious nature of any food-drug, drug-drug combinations.

Neuroleptic Malignant Syndrome (NMS)

A serious and potentially fatal syndrome caused by antipsychotics and other drugs that block dopamine receptors. Important not to allow client to become *dehydrated* (predisposing factor). More common in warm climates, in summer. Possible genetic predisposition.

Signs and Symptoms

- Fever: 103°–105° F or greater
- Blood pressure lability (hypertension or hypotension)
- Tachycardia (>130 bpm)
- Tachypnea (> 25 rpm)
- Agitation (respiratory distress, tachycardia)
- Diaphoresis, pallor
- Muscle rigidity (arm/abdomen like a board)
- Change in mental status (stupor to coma)
- Stop antipsychotic immediately.

🚫 **ALERT:** NMS is a medical emergency (10% mortality rate); hospitalization needed. Lab test: creatinine kinase (CK) to determine injury to the muscle. Drugs used to treat NMS include: bromocriptine, dantroline, levodopa, lorazepam.

Serotonin Syndrome

Can occur if client is taking one or more serotonergic drugs (e.g., SSRIs; also St. John's wort), especially higher doses. Do not combine SSRIs/SNRIs/clomipramine with MAOI; also tryptophan, dextromethorphan combined with MAOI can produce this syndrome.

If stopping fluoxetine (long half-life) to start an MAOI – must allow a 5-week washout period. At least 2 weeks for other SSRIs before starting an MAOI. Discontinue MAOI for 2 weeks before starting another anti-depressant or other interacting drug.

Signs and Symptoms

- Change in mental status, agitation, confusion, restlessness, flushing
- Diaphoresis, diarrhea, lethargy
- Myoclonus (muscle twitching or jerks), tremors

If serotonergic medication is not discontinued, progresses to:

- Worsening myoclonus, hypertension, rigor
- Acidosis, respiratory rhabdomyolysis

🚫 **ALERT:** Must discontinue serotonergic drug immediately. Emergency medical treatment and hospitalization needed to treat myoclonus, hypertension, and other symptoms.

Note: Refer to *Physicians' Desk Reference* or product package insert for complete drug information (dosages, indications, warnings, adverse effects, interactions, etc.) needed to make appropriate choices in the treatment of clients. Although every effort has been made to provide key information about medications and classes of drugs, such information is not and cannot be all-inclusive in a reference of this nature. Professional judgment, training, supervision, relevant references, and current drug information are critical to the appropriate selection, evaluation, monitoring, and management of clients and their medications.

Labs/Plasma Levels

Therapeutic Plasma Levels — Mood Stabilizers

- Lithium: 1.0–1.5 mEq/L (acute mania)
  0.6–1.2 mEq/L (maintenance)
  Toxic: >1.5 mEq/L
- Carbamazepine: 4–12 µg/mL
  Toxic >15 µg/mL
- Valproic acid: 50–100 µg/mL

Note: Lithium blood level should be drawn in the morning about 12 hours after last oral dose and before first morning dose.

Plasma Level/Lab Test Monitoring

- **Lithium –** Initially check serum level every 1–2 wk (for at least 2 mo), then every 3–6 mo; renal function every 6–12 mo; TFTs every year.
- **Carbamazepine –** Serum levels every 1–2 wk (at least for 2 mo); CBC and LFTs every mo, then CBCs/LFTs every 6–12 mo; serum levels every 3–6 mo as appropriate.
- **Valproic acid –** Serum level checks every 1–2 wk; CBC/LFTs every mo; serum level every 3–6 mo; CBC/LFT every 6–12 mo.

Disorders and Labs/Tests

- Labs and tests should be performed on all clients before arriving at a diagnosis to rule out a physical cause that may mimic a psychological disorder and before starting treatments. Tests should be repeated as appropriate after diagnosis to monitor treatments/reevaluate.

Disorder	Labs/Tests
Anxiety	Physical exam, psych eval, mental status exam, TFTs (hyperthyroidism), CBC, general chemistry, toxicology screens (substance use); anxiety inventories/rating scales

Continued

Disorder	Labs/Tests
Neurocognitive disorders	Physical exam, psych eval, mental status exam, Mini-Mental State Exam, TFTs, CBC, LFTs, general chemistry, toxicology screens (substance use), B_{12}, folate, UA, HIV, FTA-ABS (syphilis), depression inventories/rating scales (Geriatric Rating Scale), CT/MRI, Structural MRI (Vernuri 2010), CSF biomarkers (Andersson 2011)
Depression	Physical exam, psych eval, mental status exam, Mini-Mental State Exam (R/O dementia), TFTs (hypothyroidism), LFTs, CBC, general chemistry, toxicology screens (substance use); depression inventories/rating scales (R/O pseudodementia), CT/MRI
Mania	Physical exam, psych eval, mental status exam, Young Mania Rating Scale (bipolar I), Mood Disorder Questionnaire (see Assessment Tab), TFTs (hyperthyroidism), toxicology screens (substance use); CBC, UA, ECG (<40 y), serum levels (VA, CBZ, Li), BMI, general chemistry/metabolic panel, pregnancy test, CT/MRI
Postpartum depression	Physical exam, psych eval (history of previous depression/psychosis), mental status exam, TFTs, CBC, general chemistry, Edinburgh Postnatal Depression Scale, monitor/screen during postpartal period (fathers also)
Schizophrenia	Physical exam, psych eval, mental status exam, TFTs (hyperthyroidism), LFTs, toxicology screens (substance use), CBC, UA, serum glucose, BMI, general chemistry/metabolic panel, VeriPsych biomarker blood test (VeriPsych 2010), pregnancy test, CT/MRI; Positive and Negative Syndrome Scale, AIMS

Clozaril Protocol – Clozaril Patient Management System

Indications for use: Patients with a diagnosis of schizophrenia, unresponsive or intolerant to *three* different neuroleptics from at least *two* different therapeutic groups, when given adequate doses for adequate duration.

- System for monitoring WBCs of patients on clozapine. Important because of possible (life-threatening) agranulocytosis and leukopenia.
- Need to monitor WBCs, absolute neutrophil count (ANC), and differential
- WBC and ANC weekly first 6 mo, then bi-weekly, then weekly for 1 month after discontinuation.

- Only available in 1-wk supply (requires WBCs, patient monitoring, and controlled distribution through pharmacies).
- If WBC <3000 mm^3 or granulocyte count <1500 mm^3 — withhold clozapine (monitor for signs & symptoms of infection).
- Monthly monitoring approved under certain situations (FDA approval 2005).
- Patients must be registered with the Clozaril National Registry (see www.clozaril.com).

Psychotropic Drugs A – Z

The following drugs are listed alphabetically within this tab by generic name (example trade name in parentheses):

*Latest drugs approved/released into the marketplace.

NOTE: Access 78 complete psychotropic drug monographs online at DavisPlus: http://davisplus.fadavis.com. Keyword: Pedersen

Psychotropic Drugs A – Z (Alphabetical Listing)

Psychotropic Drug Tables that follow include each drug's half life (T½), protein binding, pregnancy categories, Canadian drug trade names (*in italics*), dose ranges and adult doses, most common side effects (CSE), geriatric and dose considerations, and LIFE-THREATENING (ALL CAPS) side effects, listed alphabetically by generic name. *(See Alert at end of tab as well as FDA Warnings.)*

Generic (Trade)	Dose Range/ Adult Daily Dose	Use/Common Side Effects (CSE)	Geriatric & Dose Considerations	Classification Assessment Cautions
Alprazolam (Xanax, Xanax *(anxiety); panic:* Novo-Alprazol, Nu-Alpraz) Intermediate T½ = 12–15 h Pregnancy category D	0.25–0.5 mg po 2–3 times daily *(anxiety); panic:* 0.5 mg 3 times daily; not to exceed 10 mg/d; XR: 0.5–1 mg once daily in AM: usual range 3–6 mg/d	*Use:* Anxiety; panic; *unlabeled:* PMS CSE: Dizziness, drowsiness, lethargy; sometimes confusion, hangover, paradoxical excitation, diarrhea, nausea, vomiting	↓ Dose required; begin 0.25 mg 2–3 times/d; assess renal function in long-term therapy; avoid grapefruit juice; risk for falls Elderly have ↑ sensitivity to CNS and risk for benzodiazepines.	Antianxiety agent Monitor CBC, liver, renal function in long-term therapy; risk for psychological/ physical dependence; seizures on abrupt discontinuation. Interacts with alcohol, anti-depressants, antihistamines, other benzos, and opioids.

Psychotropic Drugs A – Z (Alphabetical Listing)—cont'd

Generic (Trade)	Dose Range/ Adult Daily Dose	Use/Common Side Effects (CSE)	Geriatric & Dose Considerations	Classification Assessment Cautions
Amitriptyline (Elavil, Apo-*Amitriptyline*) $T\frac{1}{2}$ = 10–50 h Protein binding = >95% Pregnancy category C	Range: 50–300 mg/d; dosage: 75 mg/d po in divided doses up to 150 mg/d or 50–100 mg hs; increase by 25–50 mg to 150 mg (in hospital: start 100 mg/d up to 300 mg)	*Use:* Depression; *unlabeled:* chronic pain *CSE:* Blurred vision, dry eyes, dry mouth, sedation, hypotension, constipation, ARRHYTHMIAS	Use caution: Orthostatic hypotension, sedation, confusion (falls); CV disease; titrate slowly	Antidepressant [TCA] Hx CV disease or high doses: *Monitor* ECG prior to and through Rx

Continued

Psychotropic Drugs A – Z (Alphabetical Listing)—cont'd

Generic (Trade)	Dose Range/ Adult Daily Dose	Use/Common Side Effects (CSE)	Geriatric & Dose Considerations	Classification Assessment Cautions
Aripiprazole (Abilify, Abilify Discmelt, Abilify Oral Solution and Injection, Ability Maintena [once-monthly extended-release IM: 400 mg monthly)) T½ = 75 h; dehydroaripi- prazole = 94 h Protein binding = >99% T½ = 2–3 h Pregnancy category C	*Schizophrenia:* 10–15 mg/d po (up to 30 mg/d); ↑ (man c/mixed) 2 wk at a given dose. *Bipolar I (acute manic/mixed):* start 15 mg/d (up to 30 mg/d) *Agitation* (schizophrenia or bipolar): *IM* – 9.75 mg; range 5.25–15 mg See Prescribing info for adjunct Rx	*Use:* Schizophrenia, acute bipolar mania, augmentation of antide- pressant therapy; Autistic irritability; *IM:* Agitation (bipolar/ schizophrenia) *CSE:* Nausea, anxiety, confusion, constipation, orthostat- ic hypotension, ↑ salivation, ecchymoses, NMS	Orthostatic hypotension; *Contraindicated:* dis:ase; ↑ mortality in elderly with dementia-related psychosis	Antipsychotic [Atypical] *Contraindicated:* Lactation; caution with CV/cere- brovascular diseases; avoid dehydration; NEUROLEPTIC MALIGNANT SYNDROME *Monitor* BMI, FBS, and lipids

Continued

Psychotropic Drugs A – Z (Alphabetical Listing)—cont'd

Generic (Trade)	Dose Range/ Adult Daily Dose	Use/Common Side Effects (CSE)	Geriatric & Dose Considerations	Classification Assessment Cautions
Asenapine (Saphris) T½ = 24 h Protein binding = 95% Sublingual (SL) Pregnancy category C	*Schizophrenia (acute):* 5 mg SL twice daily; *maintenance:* start 5 mg SL twice daily X 1 wk, to 10 mg SL twice daily *Bipolar mania (monotherapy):* start 10 mg SL twice daily to 5–10 mg SL twice daily; *adjunct to lithium/valproate:* 5 mg twice daily to 5–10 mg twice daily; maximum dose: 10 mg twice daily	*Use: Schizophrenia,* acute and maintenance; *Bipolar I,* acute mania and mixed episodes; and adjunctive therapy with lithium or valproate *CSE: schizophrenia:* akathisia, somnolence, oral hypoesthesia *Bipolar:* somnolence, dizziness, EPS other than akathisia, weight gain	Caution in elderly because of orthostatic hypotension, dizziness, or somnolence. Start at lowest dose. Only 1.1% of clinical trial patients were >65. *Warning:* ↑mortality in elderly with dementia-related psychosis	Antipsychotic [Atypical] *Caution:* coadministration w *fluvoxamine* (strong CYP1A2 inhibitor) *and paroxetine* (CYP2D6 substrate and inhibitor); No adjustment needed for renal impairment, do not use with severe hepatic impairment. Caution with alcohol, other centrally acting drugs, and antihypertensive agents. *Assess:* Monitor for suicidality early on and throughout Rx. TD, NMS, DM, orthostatic hypotension, QT prolongation, seizures

Continued

Psychotropic Drugs A – Z (Alphabetical Listing)—cont'd

Generic (Trade)	Dose Range/ Adult Daily Dose	Use/Common Side Effects (CSE)	Geriatric & Dose Considerations	Classification Assessment Cautions
Benztropine (Cogentin, *Apo-Benztropine*) T½ = Unknown Pregnancy category C	*Parkinsonism:* 0.5–6 mg/d *EPS:* PO/IM/IV: 1–4 mg qd or 1–2 mg po bid or 2–3 times daily; *acute dystonia:* IM/IV: 1–2 mg po bid	*Use:* Parkinson's, drug-induced EPS, and acute dystonia *CSE:* Blurred vision, dry mouth, dry eyes, constipation, urinary retention	*Use cautiously:* ↑ risk of adverse reactions	**Antiparkinson agent** *Contraindicated:* Narrow-angle glaucoma and TD; Assess parkinsonian/ EPS symptoms; Assess bowel function (constipation)/ urinary retention *IM/IV:* Monitor pulse/ BP closely; advise slow position changes
Bupropion HCL (Wellbutrin, Wellbutrin SR, Wellbutrin XL, Forfivo XL [once daily]) Bupropion hydro-bromide (Aplenzin) [Once daily dosing] T½ = 14 h Pregnancy category B	*IR:* 100 mg po bid; after 3 d ↑ to tid; wk 4 to 450 mg/d in divided doses *Aplenzin:* 348 mg/d once in AM; start 174 mg/d, → after 4 d to *max:* 522 mg/d; *Forfivo XL:* 450 mg once daily	*Use:* Depression; adult ADHD (SR only); ↑ female sexual desire *CSE:* Agitation, headache, dry mouth, nausea, vomiting, SEIZURES	*Use cautiously;* ↑ risk of drug accumulation	**Antidepressant** *Contraindicated:* Hx bulimia or anorexia; seizure disorder Seizure risk ↑ at doses >450 mg; **avoid alcohol CAUTION:** Bupropion XL 300 (Teva) pulled off market as ineffective (2012).

Continued

Psychotropic Drugs A – Z (Alphabetical Listing)—cont'd

Generic (Trade)	Dose Range/ Adult Daily Dose	Use/Common Side Effects (CSE)	Geriatric & Dose Considerations	Classification Assessment Cautions
Buspirone (BuSpar) $T\frac{1}{2}$ = 2–3 h Protein binding = >95% Pregnancy category B	15–60 mg/d po	*Use:* Anxiety management; anxiety w depression *CSE:* Dizziness, drowsiness, blurred vision, palpitations, chest pain, nausea, rashes, myalgia, sweating	*Contraindicated:* Severe renal/ hepatic disease	Antianxiety agent *Contraindicated:* Severe renal/hepatic impairment; does not appear to cause dependence
Carbamazepine (Tegretol, Tegretol XR, Equetro, Epitol, *Apo-Carbamazepine, Tegretol CR* $T\frac{1}{2}$ = single dose = 25–65 h; chronic dosing = 8–29 h Pregnancy category D	*Start:* 200 mg/d or 100 mg bid; increase weekly by 200 mg/d until therapeutic level/ mania improvement. Equetro (Bipolar): 400 mg/d divided doses, twice daily up to 1600 mg/d	*Use:* Bipolar I: Acute mania/mixed (Equetrol); *CSE:* Ataxia, drowsiness, blurred vision. APLASTIC ANEMIA, AGRANULOCYTOSIS, THROMBOCYTOPENIA, STEVENS-JOHNSON SYNDROME (SJS)	Use cautiously; CV/hepatic disease; BPH and increased intraocular pressure	Anticonvulsant/ mood stabilizer *Caution:* Impaired liver/cardiac functions. Monitor CBC, platelets, reticulocytes. HLA-B* 1502 typing for those genetically at risk (Asians). Therapeutic Range (4–12 mg/mL). *Sx of SJS:* cough, FUO, mucosal lesions, rash; stop CBZ

Continued

Psychotropic Drugs A – Z (Alphabetical Listing)—cont'd

Generic (Trade)	Dose Range/ Adult Daily Dose	Use/Common Side Effects (CSE)	Geriatric & Dose Considerations	Classification Assessment Cautions
Chlordiazepoxide (Librium). Libritabs, Apo-Chlordiazepoxide; Librax [comb w clidinium]. Limbitrol DS [comb w amitriptyline]) T½ = 5–30 h Pregnancy category D	*Anxiety:* 5–25 mg po 3–4 × daily *Alcohol withdrawal:* IM: 50–100 mg; repeat in 3–4 h or po 50–100 mg; repeat until agitation ↓ (to 400 mg/d)	*Use:* Adjunct anxiety lo aged sedation in the elderly and is associated with ↑ risk of falls. *Contraindicated:* Narrow-angle glaucoma, porphyria; caution with hepatic/renal impairment and history of suicide attempt/substance abuse	May cause pro-longed sedation in the elderly and is associated with ↑risk of falls. *Contraindicated:* Narrow-angle glaucoma, porphyria; caution with hepatic/renal impairment and history of suicide attempt/substance abuse	Antianxiety agent [benzo] *Contraindicated:* Narrow-angle glaucoma. Must reduce dose or consider short-acting benzodi-azpine
Chlorpromazine (Thorazine, Thor-Prom, Largactil, Novo-Chlorpromazine/ T½ = initial 2 h; end 30 h Protein binding = ≥ 90% Pregnancy category unknown	*Range:* 40–800 mg/d po *Psychoses:* 10–25 mg po 2–4 times/d; may ↑ q 3–4 d up to 1 g/d; IM: Start 25–50 mg IM to max. 400 mg q 3–12 h (max. 1 g/d)	*Use:* Psychosis; combativeness CSE: Hyctensioา (esp IM), blurred vision, sedation, constipation, drγ mouth, photosensitivity, NMS, AGRAN-U-OC¥TOSIS	*Caution:* Sedating; decrease initial dose. *Caution:* BPH	Antipsychotic [Conventional] *Contraindicated:* G aucoma, bone marrow depression, severe liver/CV disease. Monitor BP, pulse, and respirations, CBCs, LFTs, and eye exams; EPS, akathisia, NMS

Continued

Psychotropic Drugs A – Z (Alphabetical Listing)—cont'd

Generic (Trade)	Dose Range/ Adult Daily Dose	Use/Common Side Effects (CSE)	Geriatric & Dose Considerations	Classification Assessment Cautions
Citalopram (Celexa) T½ = 35 h Pregnancy category C	*Range:* 20–60 mg/d po Start 20 mg po daily, increased weekly, if needed, by 20 mg/d up to 60 mg/d (usual dose: 40 mg/d)	*Use:* Depression *CSE:* Apathy, confusion, drowsiness, insomnia, abdominal pain, anorexia, diarrhea, dyspepsia, nausea, sweating, tremor	20 mg po once daily; may increase to 40 mg/d only in those not responding. Lower doses with hepatic/renal impairment.	Antidepressant [SSRI] *Contraindicated:* Use within 14 days of MAOI; *Caution:* hx of mania or seizures; serotonin syndrome with SAMe or St. John's wort; monitor for mood changes and assess for suicide
Clomipramine (Anafranil, Apo-Clomipramine) T½ = 20–30 h Pregnancy category C	*Range:* 25–250 mg/d po Start 25 mg/d po; gradually increase to 100 mg/d (up to 250 mg/d)	*Use:* OCD *CSE:* Dizziness, drowsiness, increased appetite, weight gain, constipation, nausea	Use with caution in elderly (sedation, orthostatic hypotension; CV disease; BPH)	Antidepressant [TCA] *Caution:* CV disease including conduction abnormalities, hx: seizures, bipolar, hypotensive disorders; avoid alcohol; *fatal with MAOIs.*

Continued

Psychotropic Drugs A – Z (Alphabetical Listing)—cont'd

Generic (Trade)	Dose Range/ Adult Daily Dose	Use/Common Side Effects (CSE)	Geriatric & Dose Considerations	Classification Assessment Cautions
Clonazepam (Klonopin, Rivotril, Syn-Clonazepam) T½ = 18–50 h Schedule IV Pregnancy category D	*Range:* 1.5–4 mg/d po (panic/anxiety); as high as 6 mg/d; up to 20 mg/d for seizures	*Use:* Panic disorder, seizure disorders; rest-less leg syndrome CSE: Behavioral changes, drowsiness, ataxia	*Caut on:* Drowsiness; *Contraindicated:* Severe liver disease; assess for drowsiness; dose-related. *Monitor:* CBC/LFTs with prolonged therapy	Antianxiety agent [benzo] *Contraindicated:* Liver disease
Clozapine (Clozaril, FazaClo) T½ = 8–12 h Protein binding = 95% [FazaClo—orally disintegrating tablets] Pregnancy category B	*Range:* 300–900 mg/d po Start 25 mg po 1–2 × daily; ↑ 25–50 mg/d over 2 wk up to 300–450 mg/d (not to exceed 900 mg/d) FazaClo: start 12.5 mg 1–2 × daily; no water needed	*Use:* Refractive schizophrenia (unresponsive to other treatments) CSE: Dizziness, seda-tion, hypotension, tachycardia, constipa-tion, NMS, SEIZURES, AGRANULOCYTOSIS, LEUKOPENIA, MYOCARDITIS (D/C clozapine)	Use cautiously with CV/hepatic/rena disease; sedating; ↑ mortality in elderly with dementia-related psychosis	Antipsychotic [Atypical] *Must follow Clozari protocol:* Monitor BP/pulse; CBC (WBC/diff <3000/mm³–withhold clozapine). (See Clozaril Protocol in Drug-Lab tab) *Monitor* for signs of myocarditis akathisia, EPS, and NMS; also BMI, FBS, and lipids. (For FazaClo Protocol, see www.Fazaclo.com)

Psychotropic Drugs A – Z (Alphabetical Listing)—cont'd

Generic (Trade)	Dose Range/ Adult Daily Dose	Use/Common Side Effects (CSE)	Geriatric & Dose Considerations	Classification Assessment Cautions
Desipramine (Norpramin, Pertofrane) T½ = 12–27 h Protein binding = 90%–92% Pregnancy category C	*Range:* 25–300 mg/d 100–200 mg/d po single or divided doses (up to 300 mg/d)	*Use:* Depression; *unlabeled:* chronic pain *CSE:* Blurred vision, dry eyes, dry mouth, sedation, hypotension, constipation ARRHYTHMIAS	*Reduce dosage:* 25–50 mg/d po (in divided doses (up to 150 mg/d); sedation. *Caution* with CV disease, BPH; monitor BP & pulse	Antidepressant [TCA] *Contraindicated:* Narrow-angle glaucoma. *Monitor BP/* pulse; ECG prior to and through Rx if hx of CV disease or high doses

Continued

Psychotropic Drugs A – Z (Alphabetical Listing)—cont'd

Generic (Trade)	Dose Range/ Adult Daily Dose	Use/Common Side Effects (CSE)	Geriatric Assessment Considerations	Classification Assessment Cautions
Desvenlafaxine (Pristiq) T½ = 11 h Pregnancy category C	*Adults:* 50 mg po once daily; in clinical studies (50–400 mg/d) there did not seem to be additional benefit above 50 mg/d. The recommended dose with moderate renal impairment (24-hr CrCl = 30–50 mL/min) is 50 mg/d; with severe renal impairment (24-hr CrCl < 30 mL/min) or end-stage renal disease (ESRD) 50 mg every other day. *Extended release formulation* (once-daily dosing) should not be chewed or crushed	*Use:* Major depressive disorder in adults only CSE: Anxiety, dizziness, headache, abnormal dreams, insomnia, nervousness, weakness, mydriasis, rhinitis, visual disturbances, anorexia, constipation, diarrhea, dry mouth, dyspepsia, nausea, vomiting, weight loss, sexual dysfunction, ecchymoses, paresthesias, chills	*Caution* in elderly with CV disease, hypertension, liver or renal impairment, and hx of increased intraocular pressure or narrow-angle glaucoma. *Monitor* for suicidality and see dosing for renal impairment.	Antidepressant [SNRI] Concurrent MAOI therapy is contraindicated. Use with alcohol, CNS depressants not recommended. Beware of multiple drug-drug interactions; no adjustment needed for mild/ moderate hepatic. *Caution* with preexisting hypertension; hypertension dose-related. Assess: monitor for suicidality early on and throughout Rx. Also BP before/ after Rx (↓ dose or D/C). Taper slowly to D/C.

Continued

Psychotropic Drugs A – Z (Alphabetical Listing)—cont'd

Generic (Trade)	Dose Range/ Adult Daily Dose	Use/Common Side Effects (CSE)	Geriatric & Dose Considerations	Classification Assessment Cautions
Diazepam (Valium, Apo-Diazepam, Vivol) T½ = 20–50 h (up to 100 h for metabolites) Schedule IV Pregnancy category D	*Range:* 4–40 mg/d Anxiety: *po:* 2–10 mg 2–4 × daily; *IM/IV:* 2–10 mg q 4 h prn. *Alcohol WD:* po: 10 mg 3–4 × first 24 h; then 5 mg 3–4 × daily; *IM/IV:* 10 mg, then 5–10 mg in 3–4 h as needed	*Use:* Anxiety adjunct; alcohol withdrawal *CSE:* Dizziness, drowsiness, lethargy	Dosage reduction required; *caution:* hepatic/renal disease; *assess:* risk for falls; prolonged sedation in the elderly	Antianxiety agent [benzo] *Monitor:* BP/pulse/ respirations; CBC, LFTs; renal tests periodically with prolonged therapy; *Monitor for dependence. Alcoholics:* ETOH withdrawal-*assess for:* tremors, delirium, agitation, hallucinations

Continued

Psychotropic Drugs A – Z (Alphabetical Listing)—cont'd

Generic (Trade)	Dose Range/ Adult Daily Dose	Use/Common Side Effects (CSE)	Geriatric Assessment & Dose Considerations	Classification Assessment Cautions
Divalproex sodium (Depakote, Depakote ER, Epival) [Valproate] T½ = 5–20 h Pregnancy category D	*Range:* 500–1500 mg/d po (up to 4000 mg/d) *Initially:* 750 mg/d in divided doses, titrated to clinical effect/plasma levels; *ER:* Single dose at bedtime	*Use:* Bipolar, acute mania & prophylaxis *CSE:* Nausea, vomiting, indigestion HEPATOTOXICITY, PANCREATITIS	*Caution* with renal impairment, mood stabilizer *Contraindicated:* Hepatic impairment; *Monitor* LFTs, serum ammonia before and throughout Rx for excessive somnolence	Anticonvulsant/ mood stabilizer Hyperammonemia: D/C VA. *Caution:* Renal/ bleeding disorders; bone marrow depression; *teratogenicity;* need VA levels (50–100 µg/mL)

Continued

Psychotropic Drugs A – Z (Alphabetical Listing)—cont'd

Generic (Trade)	Dose Range/ Adult Daily Dose	Use/Common Side Effects (CSE)	Geriatric & Dose Considerations	Classification Assessment Cautions
Doxepin (Sinequan, Zonalon, *Triadapin*) T½ = 8–25 h Pregnancy category C	*Range:* 25–300 mg/d po 25 mg po 3 × daily, up to 150 mg (inpatient up to 300 mg/d)	*Use:* Depression/ anxiety *CSE:* Blurred vision, dry eyes, dry mouth, sedation, hypotension, constipation, ARRHYTHMIAS	*Dose reduction:* 25–50 mg/d po initially, increase as needed; *Caution* with preexisting CV disease, BPH; *assess* for falls and anticholinergic effects	Antidepressant [TCA] *Monitor* blood pressure and pulse; ECGs with hx of CV disease; WBC w diff, LFTs, and serum glucose periodically
Duloxetine (Cymbalta) T½ = 12 h Protein binding = >90% Pregnancy category C	*Range:* 40–60 mg/d; 20–30 mg po twice daily	*Use:* Major depressive disorder *CSE:* fatigue, drowsiness, insomnia, ↓ appetite, constipation, dry mouth, nausea, dysuria, ↑ sweating, SEIZURES	Use with *caution;* increase slowly	Antidepressant [SNRI] *Contraindicated:* Concurrent MAOIs, hepatic impairment/ ETOH use; with renal impairment: start with lower dose. *Monitor* BP (↑ BP dose-related) & LFTs; *monitor* for suicidality

Continued

Psychotropic Drugs A – Z (Alphabetical Listing)—cont'd

Generic (Trade)	Dose Range/ Adult Daily Dose	Use/Common Side Effects (CSE)	Geriatric Assessment & Dose Considerations	Classification Assessment Cautions
Escitalopram (Lexapro) T½ = increased in hepatic impairment Pregnancy category C	*Range:* 10–20 mg/d; 10 mg po once daily, may increase to 20 mg/d after 1 wk	*Use:* Depression, generalized anxiety disorder CSE: Insomnia, diarrhea, neusea, sexual dysfunction	↓ dose in elderly; caution with hepatic/renal impairment (10 mg po once daily); T½ increased in the elderly	Antidepressant [SSRI] *Contraindicated:* Concurrent MAOIs or citalopram *Caution:* hx mania/ seizures or risk for suicide; *monitor for suicidality*
Eszopiclone (Lunesta) T½ = 6 h Protein binding = weakly bound Schedule IV Pregnancy category C	*Range:* 1–3 mg po Start at 2 mg po hs, may↑ to 3 mg if needed	*Use:* Insomnia: Sleep latency/maintenance CSE: Anxiety, confusion, depression, headache, migraine, dizziness, hallucinations	Elderly should start with 1 mg po dose and take immediately before bedtime; sho uld not exceed 2 mg/hs	Sedative/hypnotic *Severe hepatic impairment:* Start 1 mg. *Caution:* Concomitant illness, drug/ETOH abuse, psychiatric illness, abrupt withdrawal (see FDA warning, end of tab)

Psychotropic Drugs A – Z (Alphabetical Listing)—cont'd

Generic (Trade)	Dose Range/ Adult Daily Dose	Use/Common Side Effects (CSE)	Geriatric & Dose Considerations	Classification Assessment Cautions
Fluoxetine (Prozac, Prozac Weekly, Serafem [PMDD]) T½ = 1–3 d (norfluoxetine: 5–7 d) Protein binding = 94.5% Pregnancy category C	*Range:* 20–80 mg po *Depression/OCD:* Start 20 mg/d po, may ↑ weekly up to 80 mg; *Panic disorder:* Start 10 mg/d po up to 60 mg/d; *Prozac Weekly:* 90 mg/wk *Serafem:* start 20 mg/d up to 60 mg/d or start 14 days before menstruation	*Use:* Depression (also geriatric), OCD, bulimia nervosa, panic disorder *CSE:* Anxiety, drowsiness, headache, insomnia, nervousness, diarrhea, sexual dysfunction, ↑ sweating, pruritus, tremor	*Starting dose:* 10 mg/d (not to exceed 60 mg); *Caution* with hepatic/renal impairment and with multiple medications (long T½); Elderly at risk for excessive CNS stimulation, sleep disturbances, and agitation.	Antidepressant [SSRI] Serious fatal reactions with MAOIs, long washout needed. *Caution:* Hepatic/renal/ pregnancy/seizures. *Peds/Adol (18–24 y):* May increase risk of suicidal thinking and behavior; *must closely monitor*

Continued

Psychotropic Drugs A – Z (Alphabetical Listing)—cont'd

Generic (Trade)	Dose Range/ Adult Daily Dose	Use/Common & Side Effects (CSE)	Geriatric & Dose Considerations	Classification Assessment Cautions
Fluphenazine hydrochloride (Prolixin, Apo-Fluphenazine) T½ = 4.7–15.3 h Fluphenazine decanoate (Prolixin decanoate) T½ = 6.8–9.6 d Fluphenazine Enanthate T½ = 3.7 d Protein binding ≥ 90% Pregnancy category C	Range: 1–40 mg/d Fluphenazine HCl: Start: 2.5–10 mg/d po (divided dose q 6–8 h); maintenance: 1–5 mg/d; IM: 1.25–2.5 mg q 6–8 h Decanoate: Start 12.5–25 mg IM/SC q 1–4 wk (may ↑ to 100 mg/dose)	Use: Psychotic disorders, schizophrenia, chronic schizophrenia CSE: EPS, photosensitivity, sedation tardive dyskinesia, AGRANULOCYTOSIS	Use lower doses: Fluphenazine HCl: Start with 1–2.5 mg/d po; caution with BP↓, respiratory disease, use with to ↓ disease: Contraindicated: severe liver/CV disease: Contraindicated: ↑ mortality in elderly with dementia-related psychosis	Antipsychotic [Conventional] Contraindicated: Severe liver/CV disease, use with pimozide, glaucoma, bone marrow depression Monitor BP, pulse, respiration, ECG changes, EPS, akathisia, TD, NMS (report immediately). Periodic CBCs, LFTs, eye exams

Continued

Psychotropic Drugs A – Z (Alphabetical Listing)—cont'd

Generic (Trade)	Dose Range/ Adult Daily Dose	Use/Common Side Effects (CSE)	Geriatric & Dose Considerations	Classification Assessment Cautions
Flurazepam (Dalmane, Apo-Flurazepam, Somnol) T½ = 2.3 h (active metabolite may be 30–200 h) Protein binding = 97% Schedule IV Pregnancy category X	*Range:* 15–30 mg *Usual dose:* 15–30 mg po hs	*Use:* Short-term insomnia management (<4 wk) *CSE:* Drowsiness, confusion, dizziness, paradoxical excitation, blurred vision, constipation	Initial dose ↓; 15 mg po initially hs; hepatic disease; warn patient and family about ↑ risk for falls and requires assessment for falls and fall prevention	Sedative/hypnotic [benzo] *Contraindicated:* CNS depression, narrow-angle glaucoma, pregnancy, lactation. *Caution:* Hepatic disease, hx suicide attempts, avoid alcohol (see FDA warning, end of tab)
Fluvoxamine (Luvox) T½ = 13.6–15.6 h Pregnancy category C	*Range:* 50–300 mg/d *Start:* 50 mg/d po hs, ↑ 50 mg q 4–7 d (divide equally, if dose >100 mg) (do not exceed 300 mg/d)	*Use:* OCD. *Off label:* depression, GAD, PTSD. *CSE:* Headache, dizziness, drowsiness, nervousness, insomnia, nausea, diarrhea, constipation	Reduce dose, titrate slowly; caution with impaired hepatic function	Antidepressant [SSRI] Serious fatal reactions with MAOIs. *Peds/Adol* (18–24 yl): Weigh risk vs benefit. *Monitor* closely for suicidality

Continued

Psychotropic Drugs A – Z (Alphabetical Listing)—cont'd

Generic (Trade)	Dose Range/ Adult Daily Dose	Use/Common Side Effects (CSE)	Geriatric Assessment & Dose Considerations	Classification Cautions
Gabapentin (Neurontin, Gabarone) T½ = 5–7 h Pregnancy category C	*Range:* 900–1800 mg/d *Start:* 300 mg po 3 × daily; titrate up to 1800 mg/d in divided doses (doses up to 3600 mg/d have been used)	*Use:* Partial seizures. *Off-label:* Bipolar disorder and chronic pain CSE: Drowsiness, ataxia, confusion, depression may also cause dizziness, hostility, vertigo, hypertension, anorexia	Use cautiously; especially with renal impairment (↓ dose and/or ↑ dosing interval).	Anticonvulsant/ mood stabilizer *Caution:* Renal impairment (↓ dose). Discontinuation requires at least 1 wk; should be done gradually; dosages no more than 12 h apart. Risk of CNS depression with alcohol, opioids, other CNS depressants.

Psychotropic Drugs A – Z (Alphabetical Listing)—cont'd

Generic (Trade)	Dose Range/ Adult Daily Dose	Use/Common Side Effects (CSE)	Geriatric & Dose Considerations	Classification Assessment Cautions
Haloperidol (Haldol, Apo-Haloperidol) Haloperidol decanoate T½ = 21–24 h Protein Binding = 90% Pregnancy category C	*Range:* 1–100 mg/d *Haloperidol:* 0.5–5 mg po 2–3 × d (to 100 mg/d). *Decanoate (IM):* 10–15 times the oral dose; given monthly	*Use:* Psychotic disorders, aggressive states, schizophrenia *CSE:* EPS, blurred vision, constipation, dry mouth/eyes, NMS, SEIZURES	*Dosage reduction required:* 0.5–2 mg po two × daily; increasing gradually. *Caution:* CV/ diabetes, BPH. ↑ mortality in dementia-related psychosis in the elderly.	Antipsychotic [Conventional] *Monitor* BP, pulse, respiration, akathisia, EPS, tardive dyskinesia, NMS (report immediately). Perform CBC w diff, LFTs, eye exams periodically. Avoid alcohol/CNS depressants. *Caution:* Toxic encephalopathy w haloperidol + lithium
Hydroxyzine (Atarax, Vistaril, Apo-Hydroxyzine, Novohydroxyzin) T½ = 3 h Pregnancy category C	Range: 100–400 mg/d 25–100 mg po 4 × daily (do not exceed 600 mg/d).	Use: Anxiety, pruritus, preop sedation CSE: Drowsiness, dry mouth, pain at IM site	Dosage reduction; severe hepatic disease; at ↑ risk for falls and CNS effects. *Monitor* for drowsiness, agitation, sedation.	Antianxiety/ sedative/hypnotic *Contraindicated* in pregnancy. Use cautiously in severe hepatic dysfunction. Avoid alcohol/ CNS depressants.

Continued

Psychotropic Drugs A – Z (Alphabetical Listing)—cont'd

Generic (Trade)	Dose Range/ Adult Daily Dose	Use/Common Side Effects (CSE)	Geriatric & Dose Considerations	Classification Assessment Cautions
Iloperidone (Fanapt) Protein binding = 95% Pregnancy Category C	Recommended target dosage is 12–24 mg/day administered twice daily. Start 1 mg twice daily and titrate up slowly to avoid orthostatic hypotension.	*Use:* Acute treatment of schizophrenia *CSE:* not include dizziness, dry mouth, fatigue, nasal congestion, orthostatic hypotension, somnolence, tachycardia, weight gain	Clinical trials did not include enough pts 65 y or older for comparison to younger adults. *Great caution* because of dizziness, orthostatic hypotension. *Warning:* ↑ mortality in elderly with dementia-related psychosis	*Caution:* Prolongs QT interval and may be associated with arrhythmia and sudden death—consider other antipsychotics first. Avoid use in combination with other drugs that prolong QTc. Monitor for hyperglycemia, DM, weight gain, TD, NMS, suicidality early on and throughout Rx. Beware of orthostatic hypotension, syncope. Cases of PRIAPISM have been reported. Not recommended for hepatic impairment. Beware multiple drug interactions.

Continued

Psychotropic Drugs A – Z (Alphabetical Listing)—cont'd

Generic (Trade)	Dose Range/ Adult Daily Dose	Use/Common Side Effects (CSE)	Geriatric & Dose Considerations	Classification Assessment Cautions
Imipramine (Tofranil, Apo-Imipramine) T½ = 8–16 h Protein binding = 89–95% Pregnancy category C	*Range:* 30–300 mg/d 25–50 mg po 3–4 × daily (not to exceed 300 mg/d)	*Use:* Depression *CSE:* Blurred vision, dry eyes, dry mouth, sedation, constipation, hypotension, ARRHYTHMIAS	25 mg po hs initially, up to 100 mg/d, divided doses; Use cautiously in elderly, preexisting CV disease (*monitor ECGs*), BPH	Antidepressant [TCA] *Monitor ECGs in heart disease; also BP and pulse. Contraindicated:* Concurrent MAOIs; avoid use with SSRIs, or clonidine
Lamotrigine (Lamictal) T½ = 25.4 h (on lamotrigine alone) Pregnancy category C	*Range:* 75–250 mg/d Bipolar pt not on CBZ/VA: Start 25 mg/d po × 2 wk, then 50 mg/d × 2 wk, then 100 mg/d × 1 wk, then 200 mg/d	*Use:* Partial seizures, bipolar I disorder maintenance *CSE:* Nausea, vomiting, dizziness, headache, ataxia photosensitivity, rash, STEVENS-JOHNSON SYNDROME (SJS)	May cause dizziness/ drowsiness; *Caution* with impaired renal/CV/ hepatic disease	Anticonvulsant/ mood stabilizer *Contraindicated: Lactation. Caution:* Impaired renal/ cardiac/hepatic function, hx rash on lamotrigine. Avoid abrupt discontinuation. *Assess* for skin rash. **Sx of SJS:** Cough, FUO, mucosal lesions, rash; ***stop lamotrigine***

Continued

Psychotropic Drugs A – Z (Alphabetical Listing)—cont'd

Generic (Trade)	Dose Range/ Adult Daily Dose	Use/Common Side Effects (CSE)	Geriatric & Dose Considerations	Classification Assessment Cautions
Lithium (Eskalith, Eskalith CR, Lithobid, Lithonate, Lithotabs, Carbolith, Duralith) T½ = 20–27 h Pregnancy category D	*Acute mania:* 1800–2400 mg/d; *Maintenance:* 300–1200 mg/d. *Start:* 300–600 mg po 3 × daily; usual maintenance: 300 mg 3–4 × daily. *Slow release:* 200–300 mg po 3 × daily to start, up to 1800 mg/d (divided doses); *Extended release:* 300–600 mg po 3 × daily to start	*Use:* Bipolar disorder: Acute manic episodes; prophylaxis against recurrence *CSE:* Fatigue, headache, impaired memory, ECG changes, bloating, diarrhea, nausea, leukocytosis, polyuria, acne, hypothyroidism, tremors, weight gain, SEIZURES, ARRHYTHMIAS	*Use:* Bipolar disorder: Acute manic episodes; prophylaxis against recurrence *Initial dose* reduction recommended; *caution* w CV/renal/ thyroid disease, diabetes mellitus	Antimanic/mood stabilizer Serum lithium levels: *Acute mania:* 1.0–1.5 mEq/L; *Maintenance:* 0.6–1.2 mEq/L. Narrow therapeutic range; *Signs of toxicity:* vomiting, diarrhea, drowsiness, slurred speech, ↓ coordination. Li ↓ thyroid function (hypothyroidism)/ renal changes. *Monitor* thyroid/ kidney function, WBC w diff, electrolytes, glucose, ECG, weight (also BMI). *Caution:* Toxic encephalopathy w haloperidol + lithium

Continued

Psychotropic Drugs A – Z (Alphabetical Listing)—cont'd

Generic (Trade)	Dose Range/ Adult Daily Dose	Use/Common Side Effects (CSE)	Geriatric & Dose Considerations	Classification Assessment Cautions
Lorazepam (Ativan, Apo-Lorazepam) T½ = 10–16 h Schedule IV Pregnancy category D	*Range:* 2–6 mg/d (up to 10 mg/d); 1–3 mg po 2–3 × daily; *Insomnia:* 2–4 mg po hs	*Use:* Anxiety, insomnia *CSE:* Dizziness, drowsiness, lethargy; rapid IV: APNEA, CARDIAC ARREST	Dosage reduction; *Caution:* Hepatic/ renal/pulmonary impairment; more susceptible to CNS effects and increased risk for falls	Antianxiety/sedative/ hypnotic [benzo] *Contraindicated:* Comatose or CNS depression, pregnancy, lactation, glaucoma. *Caution:* In hepatic/renal/ pulmonary impairment/drug abuse

Continued

Psychotropic Drugs A – Z (Alphabetical Listing)—cont'd

Generic (Trade)	Dose Range/ Adult Daily Dose	Use/Common Side Effects (CSE)	Geriatric & Dose Considerations	Classification Assessment Cautions
Loxapine (Loxitane, Loxapac; New: Adasuve Inhalant) T½ = 5 h/ 12–19 h Pregnancy category C	*Range:* 20–250 mg/d *Start:* 10 mg po 2 × daily, ↑ until psychotic symptom improvement. *Acute agitation in Bipolar I or schizophrenia patient.* 10 mg in a single-use inhaler. Only 1 dose in 24 h. Only dose administered by "enrolled health care facilities."	*Use:* Schizophrenia (second line Rx); *Adasuve Inhalant:* Acute agitation in Bipolar I and schizophrenic adults. *Off label:* Other psychotic disorders, bipolar. CSE: Drowsiness, orthostatic hypotension, ataxia, constipation, nausea, blurred vision. *Adasuve Inhalation:* CSE: Unpleasant taste, sedation, throat irritation; *Black box warning:* BRONCHOSPASM. Screen for contraindications: asthma, COPD, wheezing	*Evaluate/monitor* for confusion, [Conventional] *Contraindicated:* orthostatic hypotension, ↓ dose; sedation, ↓ dose; at risk for falls; ↑ mortality in elcerly with dementia-related psychosis	Antipsychotic [Conventional] *Contraindicated:* Severe CNS depression/coma. *Caution:* Parkinson's, bone marrow suppression, cardiac, renal, respiratory disease; sedating. *Monitor* for EPS, NMS, TD, BMI, FBS, lip ds

Continued

Psychotropic Drugs A – Z (Alphabetical Listing)—cont'd

Generic (Trade)	Dose Range/ Adult Daily Dose	Use/Common Side Effects (CSE)	Geriatric & Dose Considerations	Classification Assessment Cautions
Lurasidone HCL (Latuda) T½ = 18 h Protein binding = 99% Pregnancy category B	Starting dose 40 mg po once daily, up to 80 mg once daily; take with food	*Use:* Schizophrenia *CSE:* Somnolence, akathisia, nausea, parkinsonism, agitation	*Caution:* Start with lowest dose; *monitor* for somnolence, dizziness, hypotension, cognitive/motor impairment *Warning:* ↑ mortality in elderly with dementia-related psychosis	Antipsychotic [Atypical] *Caution:* Do not use in combination w strong CYP3A4 inhibitors (keto-conazole) or inducers (rifampin). Adjust dose for moderate CYP3A4 inhibitors (dilti-azem). *Monitor* for hyperglycemia, DM, weight gain. Beware of orthosta-tic hypotension, syncope, seizures. Renal/hepatic impairment: adjust dose. *Monitor* for suicidality early on and throughout Rx.

Continued

Psychotropic Drugs A – Z (Alphabetical Listing)—cont'd

Generic (Trade)	Dose Range/ Adult Daily Dose	Use/Common Side Effects (CSE)	Geriatric Assessment & Dose Considerations	Classification Assessment Cautions
Mirtazapine (Remeron, Remeron Soltabs) T½ = 20–40 h Protein binding = 85% Pregnancy category C	*Range:* 15–45 mg/d *Start:* 15 mg/d po hs, increase q 1–2 wk up to 45 mg/d	*Use:* Major depressive disorder; *Off label:* Panic disorder, GAD, PTSD *CSE:* Drowsiness, constipation, dry mouth, increased appetite, weight gain	Lower dose; use cautiously w hepatic/renal disease	Antidepressant [~tetracyclic] *Contraindicated:* Concurrent MAOI therapy; *caution w* hx seizures, suicide attempt. Closely *monitor* for suicidality/safety nct determined in children, lactation, pregnancy. Periodic CBCs, LFTs.
Molindone (Moban) T½ = 1.5 h Pregnancy category unknown	*Range:* 15–225 mg/d *Start:* 50–75 mg/d po, increase at 3-4 d intervals (up to 225 mg)	*Use:* Psychotic disorders, schizophrenia *CSE:* Sedation, drowsiness, constipation, weight gain, blurred vision	Init in ↓ dose; *Caution w* diabetes, BPH, respiratory disease; increased risk for falls (sedation/ orthostatic hypotension); ↑ mortality in dementia-related psychosis	Antipsychotic *Contraindicated w* CNS depression. *Monitor* for EPS, NMS, and TD. *Caution* with cardiac, renal, hepatic, respiratory disease. *Monitor* for BMI, FBS, and lipids.

Continued

Psychotropic Drugs A – Z (Alphabetical Listing)—cont'd

Generic (Trade)	Dose Range/ Adult Daily Dose	Use/Common Side Effects (CSE)	Geriatric & Dose Considerations	Classification Assessment Cautions
MAOIs: Phenelzine (Nardil) Tranylcypromine (Parnate) Isocarboxazid (Marplan) T½ = Unknown [See selegiline patch] Pregnancy category C	**Phenelzine:** *Range:* 45–90 mg/d *Start:* 15 mg po 3 × daily and increase to 60–90 mg/d. **Tranylcypromine:** *Range:* 30–60 mg/d *Start:* 30 mg/d po divided dose (AM/PM) up to 60 mg/d. **Isocarboxazid:** *Range:* 20–60 mg/d *Start:* 10 mg/d po, increasing every few days (up to 60 mg/d in 2–4 divided doses)	*Use:* Atypical depression, panic disorder; other Rx ineffective or not tolerated *CSE:* Dizziness, headaches, insomnia, restlessness, blurred vision, arrhythmias, orthostatic hypotension, diarrhea, SEIZURES, HYPERTENSIVE CRISIS	Use cautiously, titrate slowly, ↑ risk of adverse reactions	Antidepressant Potentially fatal reactions with other antidepressants (SSRIs, TCAs, etc). 5-wk washout w fluoxetine. *Must follow MAOI diet (foods high in tyramine) to avoid hypertensive crisis (emergency)* [See MAOI diet in Drug-Lab tab]; hypertensive crisis from caffeine; also amphetamines, levadopa, dopamine, epinephrine, reserpine, and others. Avoid opioids (meperidine).

Continued

Psychotropic Drugs A – Z (Alphabetical Listing)—cont'd

Generic (Trade)	Dose Range/ Adult Daily Dose	Use/Common Side Effects (CSE)	Geriatric & Dose Considerations	Classification Assessment Cautions
Nadolol (Corgard; Syn-Nadolol) T½ = 10–24 h Pregnancy category C	40 mg/d po (up to 240 mg)	*Use:* Tremors, akathisia *CSE:* Fatigue, impotence, ARRYTHMIAS, CHF, BRADYCARDIA, PULMONARY EDEMA	In tial dose reduction re:ommended; d :reases in:reased se:sitiv ty to b adycardia, heart b ock, etc.); *renal impairment:* ↑ dosing intervals	Antianginal; beta b ocker *Contraindicated:* CV d seases (CHF, beta blockers
Nefazodone (Serzone*) Pregnancy category C *Withdrawn from North American market	200–600 mg/d po	*Use:* Depression *CSE:* Insomnia dizziness, drowsiness, HEPATIC FAILURE; HEPATIC TOXICITY	Initiate lower dcse; HEPATIC FAILURE; HEPATIC TOXICITY	Antidepressant Serzone has been withdrawn from tłe North American market for rare but serious liver failure; generic is still available

Continued

Psychotropic Drugs A – Z (Alphabetical Listing)—cont'd

Generic (Trade)	Dose Range/ Adult Daily Dose	Use/Common Side Effects (CSE)	Geriatric & Dose Considerations	Classification Assessment Cautions
Nortriptyline (Pamelor, Aventyl) T½ = 18–28 h Protein binding = 92% Pregnancy category D	*Range:* 75–150 mg/d po *Start:* 25 mg po 3–4 × daily up to 150 mg/d	*Use:* Major depressive disorder; *Off label:* Chronic neurogenic pain, anxiety, insomnia *CSE:* Drowsiness, fatigue, blurred vision, dry eyes/mouth, hypotension, constipation, ARRYTHMIAS	*Susceptible to side effects:* ↓ Dose: 30–50 mg/d po in divided doses; *Caution w* BPH, CV disease; *Monitor* ECGs in elderly.	Antidepressant [TCA] *Contraindicated* in narrow-angle glaucoma. Potential fatal reaction with MAOIs. *Monitor* ECGs w heart disease.
Olanzapine (Zyprexa, Zyprexa Zydis, Zyprexa Intramuscular) T½ = 21–54 h Protein binding = 93% Pregnancy category C [Zyprexa Relprevv: Extended release IM; up to 4 wk]	*Range:* 5–20 mg/d **Schizophrenia:** *Start:* 5–10 mg po/d (not to exceed 20 mg/d) **Bipolar:** *Start:* 10–15 mg/d po (not to exceed 20 mg/d); *IM (acute agitation):* 5–10 mg, may repeat in 2 h/4 h	*Use:* Schizophrenia, psychotic disorders; Bipolar: Acute mania; mixed episodes; long-term maintenance *CSE:* Agitation, dizziness, sedation, orthostatic hypotension, constipation, weight gain, NMS, SEIZURES	Dosage reduction may be needed; reduce dosage for debilitated or non-smoking females ≥65: *start at* 5 mg/d po. *Caution w* CV, CVA, BPH, hepatic disease. ↑ mortality in elderly with dementia-related psychosis	Antipsychotic [Atypical] *Monitor* for treatment-emergent diabetes (serum glucose, BMI), akathisia, EPS, NMS; perform CBCs, LFTs, eye exams. *Monitor* BP, pulse, respiratory rate, ECG.

Continued

Psychotropic Drugs A – Z (Alphabetical Listing)—cont'd

Generic (Trade)	Dose Range/ Adult Daily Dose	Use/Common Side Effects (CSE)	Geriatric & Dose Considerations	Classification Assessment Cautions
Olanzapine and fluoxetine HCl (Symbyax) Olanzapine T½ = 21–54 h Protein binding = 93% Fluoxetine T½ = 1–3 d (norfluoxetine: 5–7 d) Protein binding = 94.5% Pregnancy category C	*Dosing options:* 6/25, 6/50, 12/25, 12/50 mg/d *Efficacy:* fluoxetine 6–12 mg and olanzapine 25–50 mg. Start 6/25 mg once daily po in evening	*Use:* Bipolar depressive disorder *CSE:* Drowsiness, weight gain, dry mouth, diarrhea, increased appetite, tremor, sore throat, weakness, NMS, TD	Start with 6/25 mg/d, especially if hypotensive or hepatic impairment or slow metabolism; ↑ mortality in dementia-related psychosis in the elderly	Antipsychotic/ antidepressant Same as olanzapine and fluoxetine

Continued

Psychotropic Drugs A – Z (Alphabetical Listing)—cont'd

Generic (Trade)	Dose Range/ Adult Daily Dose	Use/Common Side Effects (CSE)	Geriatric & Dose Considerations	Classification Assessment Cautions
Oxazepam (Serax, Apo-Oxazepam) T½ = 5–15 h Protein binding = 97% Schedule IV Pregnancy category D	*Range:* 30–120 mg/d *Anxiety:* 10–30 mg po 3–4 × daily *Sedative/ alcohol withdrawal:* 15–30 mg po 3–4 × daily	*Use:* Anxiety, alcohol withdrawal *CSE:* Dizziness, drowsiness, hangover, impaired memory, blurred vision, constipation, nausea	↓ *dose:* Start 5 mg po 1–2 × daily, may increase as needed; caution w hepatic; severe COPD disease; ↑ risk for falls	Antianxiety/ sedative/hypnotic [benzo] *Contraindicated:* CNS depression, coma, narrow-angle glaucoma, pregnancy, lactation *Caution:* Hepatic dysfunction; monitor CBCs, LFTs, avoid alcohol
Paliperidone (Invega) Major active metabolite of risperidone Protein binding = 74% Pregnancy category C	*Range:* 3–12 mg/d Usual dose: 6 mg/d po extended-release tab in AM (once daily dosing)	*Use:* Schizophrenia *CSE:* Somnolence, orthostatic hypotension, akathisia, EPS, parkinsonism	*Caution w* decreased renal function; moderate to severe renal impairment (dose: 3 mg/d); ↑ mortality with dementia-related psychosis	Antipsychotic [Atypical] Causes ↑ in QT interval; avoid drugs that prolong QT int (e.g., quinidine). *Monitor BMI, FBS, and lipids.*

Continued

Psychotropic Drugs A – Z (Alphabetical Listing)—cont'd

Generic (Trade)	Dose Range/ Adult Daily Dose	Use/Common Side Effects (CSE)	Geriatric & Dose Considerations	Classification Assessment Cautions
Paroxetine HCL (Paxil, Paxil CR); **paroxetine mesylate**: Pevexa T½ = 24 h Protein binding = 95% Pregnancy category D	*Range:* 10–60 mg/d; *CR:* 12.5–75 mg/d. Depression: *Start 20 mg po q AM* (may increase by 10 mg/d at week-ly intervals) *CR: Start 25 mg po once daily, may increase weekly by 1.25 mg, up to 62.5 mg/d*	*Use: Paxil/CR/Pevexa:* Depression, panic dis-order; *Paxil/Pevexa:* OCD, GAC; *Paxil:* PTSD; *Paxil CR, PMDD; Paxil/CR:* Social anxi-ety disorder. *CSE:* Anxiety, dizziness, drowsiness, dry mouth, headache, insomnia, nausea, con-stipation, diarrhea, weakness, ejaculatory disturbance, sweating, tremor	↓ *dose:* start 10 mg/d po, up to 40 mg/d; *CR:* Start 12.5 mg po daily, up to 50 mg/d. *Caution w↑hepatic, renal impairment.*	Antidepressant/ antianxiety (SSRI) *Caution:* Hepatic, re nal, seizure disorders/ pregnancy/ lactation. *Withdrawal syndrome:* Do not stop abruptly. *Peds/Adol (18–24 y):* ↑ risk for suicide; weigh risks vs ben-efits; *Closely moni-tor for suicidality* (see FDA warning, end of tab)

Continued

Psychotropic Drugs A – Z (Alphabetical Listing)—cont'd

Generic (Trade)	Dose Range/ Adult Daily Dose	Use/Common Side Effects (CSE)	Geriatric & Dose Considerations	Classification Assessment Cautions
Phenobarbital (Luminal, *Ancalixir*) T½ = 2–6 d Schedule IV Pregnancy category D	*Range:* 30–320 mg/d *Sedation:* 30–120 mg/d po/IM (divided doses) *Hypnotic:* 120–320 mg hs (PO, SC, IV, IM)	*Use:* Sedative/ hypnotic (short term) *CSE:* Hangover, drowsiness, excitation	Use cautiously; ↓ dose; hepatic/ renal disease.	Sedative/hypnotic [Barbiturate] *Life-threatening side effects:* ANGIOEDEMA, SERUM SICKNESS, LARYNGOSPASM (IV). *IV:* Monitor BP, pulse, respiratory status. Resuscitation equipment available.
Pimozide (Orap) T½ = 29–111 h Protein binding = 99% Pregnancy category C	*Range:* 2–10 mg/d Start 1–2 mg/d po, increase as needed every other day	*Use:* Tourette's, psychosis (2nd line Rx) *CSE:* Orthostatic hypotension, palpitations, QT prolongation, drowsiness, dizziness, blurred vision	Moderately sedating; *caution in* Parkinson's, arrhythmias, cerebrovascular, cardiovascular disease; may cause orthostatic hypotension; ↑ mortality in elderly with dementia-related psychosis	Antipsychotic [Conventional] *Contraindicated:* CNS depression, prolonged QT syndrome, dysrhythmias. *Caution in* respiratory, CV, hepatic, renal disease. *Assess for* EPS, TD, akathisia, NMS, BMI, FBS, and lipids.

Continued

Psychotropic Drugs A – Z (Alphabetical Listing)—cont'd

Generic (Trade)	Dose Range/ Adult Daily Dose	Use/Common Side Effects (CSE)	Geriatric & Dose Considerations	Classification Assessment Cautions
Propranolol (Inderal, Apo-propranolol) $T_{1/2}$ = 3.4–6 h Protein binding = 93% Pregnancy category C	Tremors: 80–120 mg/d po (up to 320 mg/d) Akathisia: 30–120 mg/d po	Use: Essential tremor, anxiety, akathisia CSE: Fatigue, weakness, impotence, ARRHYTHMIAS, BRADYCARDIA, CHF, PULMONARY EDEMA	↓ dose (elderly have increased sensitivity to be a blockers); renal, hepatic, bradycardia, pulmonary disease, diabetes	Antianginal/beta blocker Contraindicated: Heart block, CHF, bradycardia. Monitor BP, pulse, & for orthostatic hypotension. Abrupt withdrawal: life-threatening arrythmias.

Continued

Psychotropic Drugs A – Z (Alphabetical Listing)—cont'd

Generic (Trade)	Dose Range/ Adult Daily Dose	Use/Common Side Effects (CSE)	Geriatric & Dose Considerations	Classification Assessment Cautions
Quetiapine (Seroquel) T½ = 6 h [Seroquel XR— once daily dosing] Pregnancy category C	Range: 150–800 mg/d *Schizophrenia:* Start 25 mg po 2 × daily, gradually increase to 300–400/800 mg/d. *Bipolar mania:* Start 100 mg/d po 2 divided doses, up to 800 mg/d (incremental) *Bipolar depression:* Start 50 mg, up to 300 mg by day 4.	*Use:* Schizophrenia, Bipolar I mania: (monotherapy and adjunct to lithium/ divalproex (bipolar maintenance); *Bipolar I and II:* acute depressive episodes *CSE:* Dizziness, headache, somnolence, weight gain, NMS, SEIZURES	May require dose reduction; use cautiously in Alzheimer's, pts ≥65 y, & hx seizures. *Warning:* ↑ mortality in elderly with dementia-related psychosis. Also *caution w CV/ hepatic disease.*	Antipsychotic [Atypical/mood stabilizer *Contraindicated:* Lactation. Caution in CV disease; cerebrovascular disease, dehydration. NMS. *Monitor* for EPS, NMS. *Monitor BP* (hypotension), pulse during dose titration. [See product prescribing info for dosing for adjunctive therapies.]

Continued

Psychotropic Drugs A – Z (Alphabetical Listing)—cont'd

Generic (Trade)	Dose Range/ Adult Daily Dose	Use/Common Side Effects (CSE)	Geriatric Assessment & Dose Considerations	Classification Assessment Cautions
Ramelteon (Rozerem) [melatonin receptor agonist] $T\frac{1}{2}$ = 1–2.6 h; M-II metabolite 2–5 h Protein binding = 82% Pregnancy category C	*Adult dose:* 8 mg po within 30 min of sleep; do not administer with high-fat meal	*Use:* Insomnia (difficulty with sleep onset) CSE: Somnolence, dizziness, nausea, fatigue, headache *FDA warning:* Risk of severe allergic reaction and complex sleep-related behaviors (e.g., sleep-driving)	As with any drug that causes somnolence and dizziness, use with caution	Sedative/hypnotic *Contraindicated:* Severe liver disease and fluvoxamine (CYP 1A2 inhibitor). *Interactions* with rifampin and azole artifungals (keto-conazole). Effect on reproductive hormones in adults (↓ testosterone, ↑ pro-lactin). Avoid alco-hol. In pregnancy, benefit must out-weigh risk. *Report:* ↓ menses, ↓ ga actorrhea, ↓ lib do, ↓ fertility.

Continued

Psychotropic Drugs A – Z (Alphabetical Listing)—cont'd

Generic (Trade)	Dose Range/ Adult Daily Dose	Use/Common Side Effects (CSE)	Geriatric & Dose Considerations	Classification Assessment Cautions
Risperidone (Risperdal, Risperdal M-Tab, Risperdal Consta Long-acting Injection) *T½ = Metabolizers:* 3 h (9-hydroxy-risperidone, 21 h) *Poor metabolizers:* 20 h (9-hydroxy-risperidone, 30 h) Pregnancy category C	*Range:* 4–12 mg/d Dosing may be once/d (↑ risk of EPS w dose > 6 mg) *Schizophrenia:* Start 1 mg po 2 × daily, ↑ to 3 mg 2 × daily (up to 16 mg/d). *IM:* 25 mg q 2 wk. may ↑ 37.5/50 mg. *Bipolar Mania:* 2–3 mg/d po (range: 1–5 mg/d)	*Use:* Schizophrenia; bipolar: mania, acute or mixed; new indication: irritability associated with autism *CSE:* EPS (akathisia), dizziness, aggression, insomnia, sedation, dry mouth, pharyngitis, cough, visual disturbances, itching, skin rash, constipation, diarrhea, libido, weight gain/loss, NMS	*Warning:* ↑ mortality in elderly with dementia-related psychosis *Caution:* Renal/hepatic disease/CV disease. *Bipolar mania:* Start 0.5 mg po 2 × daily, up to 1.5 mg 2 × daily (gradually increase weekly if necessary at small increments)	Antipsychotic [Atypical] *Caution:* Renal/hepatic impairment. Dosing may be once daily or bid and increments should be small (1 mg). Maximal effect seen with 4–8 mg/d, and doses above 6 mg/d not more efficacious, and with ↑ risk of EPS. *Monitor* BP, pulse during titration; may cause tachycardia, hypotension, QT prolongation. Establish oral dosing tolerance before using IM. *Monitor* BMI, FBS, and lipids.

Continued

Psychotropic Drugs A – Z (Alphabetical Listing)—cont'd

Generic (Trade)	Dose Range/ Adult Daily Dose	Use/Common Side Effects (CSE;	Geriatric Assessment & Dose Considerations	Classification Assessment Cautions
Selegiline Patch (Emsam) [MAOI] First transdermal patch delivering medication systemically over 24 h period. Protein binding = 90% over a 2–500 ng/mL concentration range. Pregnancy category C	Range: 6 mg/24 h to 12 mg/24 h Recommended starting and target dose: 6 mg/24 h	Use: Major depressive disorder CSE: Mild skin reaction/redness at patch site. D/C if redness continues for several hours after patch removal; hypotension, HYPERTENSION	Patients 50 yr and older at higher risk for rash	Antidepressant With doses above 6 mg/24 h, must follow MAOI diet (foods high in tyramine). Hypertensive crisis is an emergency. Contraindicated: Amphetamines, pseudoephedrine, etc; other selegiline products (Eldepryl). Monitor BP, also for headache, nausea, stiff neck, palpitations. Close monitoring of children for suicidality. Read full prescribing information.

Psychotropic Drugs A – Z (Alphabetical Listing)—cont'd

Generic (Trade)	Dose Range/ Adult Daily Dose	Use/Common Side Effects (CSE)	Geriatric & Dose Considerations	Classification Assessment Cautions
Sertraline (Zoloft) T½ = 24 h Protein binding = 98% Pregnancy category C	*Range:* 50–200 mg/d *Depression/OCD:* Start: 50 mg/d po AM or PM, may ↑ slowly/weekly to 200 mg/d *Panic disorder:* Start: 25 mg/d po, up to 50 mg/d *PTSD/SAD:* Start: 25 mg/d po (to 200 mg/d)	*Use:* Depression, panic disorder, OCD, PTSD, social anxiety disorder (SAD), PMDD; *Off label:* GAD *CSE:* Drowsiness, dizziness, fatigue, insomnia, nausea, diarrhea, dry mouth, sexual dysfunction, sweating, tremor	Caution with drowsiness, hepatic/renal impairment; start with lower dose.	Antidepressant [SSRI] *Contraindicated:* Concurrent Pimozide or MAOIs (serious fatal reactions), need 14 d washout period. Do not use with St. John's wort or SAMe. *Caution:* Hepatic/renal/ pregnancy/lactation/seizures/hx mania. *Peds/Adol:* *May increase the risk of suicidal thinking and behavior and must be closely monitored.*

Continued

Psychotropic Drugs A – Z (Alphabetical Listing)—cont'd

Generic (Trade)	Dose Range/ Adult Daily Dose	Use/Common Side Effects (CSE)	Geriatric & Dose Considerations	Classification Assessment Cautions
Thioridazine* (Mellaril, Mellaril-S, Apo-thioridazine, Novo-Ridazine) T½ = 21–24 h Protein binding = ≥90% Pregnancy category C [*Mellaril discontinued worldwide for serious side effects; generic still available]	Range: 150–800 mg/d Start: 50–100 mg po tid, increase gradually up to 800 mg/d	Use: Schizophrenia CSE: Sedation, blurred vision, dry eyes, hypotension, constipation, dry mouth, photosensitivity, NMS ARRYTHMIAS QTc PROLONGATION, AGRANULOCYTOSIS	Use cautiously, at risk for EPS/CNS adverse effects. Contraindicated: ↑ risk for falls (sedation/ dehydration/ hypotension); Caution with CV disease, BPH. Be especially careful with debilitated patients: ↑ mortality in elderly with dementia-related psychos s	Antipsychotic [Conventional] Contraindicated: QTc interval >450 msec; agents that prolong QTc interval; also, narrow-angle glaucoma, bone marrow depression, severe liver or cardiovascular disease. Monitor BP, pulse, resp, and ECGs, CBCs, eye exams. Monitor for agranulocytosis; occurs between 4–10 wk of Rx. Assess for NMS, TD, akathisia.

Psychotropic Drugs A – Z (Alphabetical Listing)—cont'd

Generic (Trade)	Dose Range/ Adult Daily Dose	Use/Common Side Effects (CSE)	Geriatric & Dose Considerations	Classification Assessment Cautions
Topiramate (Topamax) T½ = 21 h Pregnancy category C	*Range:* 50–400 mg/d (maximum dose: 1600 mg/d) *Start:* 50 mg/d po, increase 50 mg/wk up to 200 mg bid	*Use:* Seizures, migraines; *Off label:* bipolar, treatment-resistant *CSE:* Dizziness, drowsiness, impaired memory/concentration, nervousness, diplopia, nystagmus, nausea, weight loss, ataxia, paresthesias, INCREASED SEIZURES, SUICIDE ATTEMPT	Adjust dose ↓ for renal/hepatic impairment. Dosage reduction recommended if CCr <70 mL/min/ 1.73 m² for adults and geriatric population	Anticonvulsant/ mood stabilizer *Contraindicated:* Lactation. *Topiramate* has not been shown to be as effective as monotherapy in bipolar disorder, may be efficacious as adjunctive treatment. Concomitant use with valproic acid associated with hyperammonemia (with or without encephalopathy). *Monitor* for alterations in LOC, cognitive function, lethargy, vomiting.

Continued

Psychotropic Drugs A – Z (Alphabetical Listing)—cont'd

Generic (Trade)	Dose Range/ Adult Daily Dose	Use/Common Side Effects (CSE)	Geriatric & Dose Considerations	Classification Assessment Cautions
Trazodone (Oleptro, Trialodine, Trazon) T½ = 5–9 h Protein binding = 89%–95% Pregnancy category C [Desyrel discontinued]	*Range:* 150–400 mg/d (hospitalized up to 600 mg/d) *Depression:* 50 mg po tid (150 mg/d), up to 400 mg/d (titrate 50 mg every 4 d. *Insomnia:* 25–100 mg hs *Oleptro:* Start 150 mg once daily; max. dose 375 mg/d	*Use:* Major depression. *Off label:* Insomnia *CSE:* Drowsiness, hypotension, dry mouth, PRIAPISM; may also experience confusion, dizziness, insomnia, nightmares, palpitations, impotence, myalgia	Reduce dose initially. *Start:* 75 mg/d po in divided doses, increase every 4 c; titrate slowly; avoid alcohol, con- comitant use with fluoxetine, opioids, and drugs that inhibit and induce the CYP3A4 enzyme system; also kava, valerian (↑ CNS depression), St. John's wort and SAMe (serotonin syndrome)	Antidepressant/ sedative PRIAPISM (pro- longed erection): Medical emergency; caution w CV, hepatic, renal disease. Observe elderly for drowsiness & hypotension; caution about slow positional changes

Continued

Psychotropic Drugs A – Z (Alphabetical Listing)—cont'd

Generic (Trade)	Dose Range/ Adult Daily Dose	Use/Common Side Effects (CSE)	Geriatric & Dose Considerations	Classification Assessment Cautions
Trihexyphenidyl (Artane, Artane Sequels, *Apo-Trihex*) $T\frac{1}{2}$ = 3.7 h Pregnancy category C	*Range:* 6–10 mg/d (up to 15 mg/d) *Start:* 1–2 mg/d po; ↑ by 2 mg every 3–5 d *Sequels (ER):* q 12 h *after* dose is determined w tabs/elixir Monitor for decreased signs & symptoms of parkinsonian syndrome: ↓ tremors/rigidity	*Use:* Parkinson's, drug-induced parkinsonism and EPS *CSE:* Dizziness, nervousness, drowsiness, blurred vision, mydriasis, dry mouth, nausea; may also experience orthostatic hypotension, tachycardia, and urinary hesitancy	*Caution w elderly:* Causes drowsiness/ dizziness (↑ risk-adverse reactions); BPH, chronic renal, hepatic, CV, pulmonary disease	Antiparkinsonian agent *Contraindicated:* Glaucoma, thyrotoxicosis, tachycardia (due to cardiac insufficiency), acute hemorrhage. Alcohol intolerance (Elixir only). Additive effects with anticholinergic drugs and CNS depressants.

Continued

Psychotropic Drugs A – Z (Alphabetical Listing)—cont'd

Generic (Trade)	Dose Range/ Adult Daily Dose	Use/Common Side Effects (CSE)	Geriatric Assessment & Dose Considerations	Classification Assessment Cautions
Venlafaxine (Effexor, Effexor XR) T½ = venlafaxine: 3–5 h; O-desmethylven- lafaxine (ODV) 9–11 h Pregnancy category C	*Range:* 75–225 mg/d; do not exceed 375 mg/d *Start:* 75 mg/d po (2–3 divided doses), up to 225 mg/d (divided doses) (do not exceed 375 mg/d). XR: 37.5–75 mg po once daily; increase q 4 d up to 225 mg	*Use:* Major depress on, general- ized anxiety disorder (XR) and social anxiety disorder (XR) *CSE:* Anxiety, abnormal dreams, dizziness, insomnia, nervousness, visual disturbances, anorexia, dry mouth, weight loss, sexual dysfunction (bruising), SEIZURES	*Use* cautiously with CV disease (hypertension); reduce dose in renal/hepatic impairment	Antidepressant [SNRI] *Caution* with preex- isting hypertension. *Monitor* blood pres- sure (risk of sus- tained hypertension [treatment emer- gent]; may be dose-related. Concurrent MAOI therapy contraindi- cated. Avoid alcohol/ CNS depressants.
Vilazodone HCl (Viibryd) T½ = 25 h Pregnancy category C	*Start:* 10 mg once daily; titrate to 40 mg/d	*Use:* Major depressive disorder *CSE:* Diarrhea, N&V, insomnia	Nc dose adjust- ments needed; possible hyponatremia	Antidepressant [SSRI]; also 5 HT₁A receptor partial agonist; caution seme as SSRIs

Continued

Psychotropic Drugs A – Z (Alphabetical Listing)—cont'd

Generic (Trade)	Dose Range/ Adult Daily Dose	Use/Common Side Effects (CSE)	Geriatric & Dose Considerations	Classification Assessment Cautions
Zaleplon (Sonata) T½ = Unknown Pregnancy category C	*Range:* 5–20 mg hs *Usual:* 10 mg po hs. Use no longer than 7–10 d	*Use:* Short-term insomnia, unable to initiate sleep *CSE:* Drowsiness, dizziness, anxiety, amnesia (see FDA warning, end of tab)	*Lower dose:* Start at 5 mg hs, to maximum of 10 mg po hs *Caution:* Mild/ moderate hepatic impairment	Sedative/hypnotic *Contraindicated:* Severe hepatic impairment. *Avoid* other CNS depressants (alcohol, opioids, kava)
Ziprasidone (Geodon) T½ = po 7h; IM 2–5 h Protein binding = 99% Pregnancy category B	*Range:* 40–160 mg/d *Schizophrenia:* Start: 20 mg po bid, up to 80 mg bid *Mania:* Start: 40 mg po bid, up to 80 mg bid; *IM:* 10–20 mg prn (up to 40 mg/d)	*Use:* Schizophrenia, bipolar (manic and mixed); *IM:* acute agitation *CSE:* Dizziness, drowsiness, restlessness, nausea, constipation, diarrhea, PROLONGED QT INTERVAL, NMS	↓ Dose in elderly. *Contraindicated:* QT prolongation, CV/ hepatic disease and CV drugs; >65 y: Alzheimer's dementia. Risk of falls. *Warning:* ↑ mortality in elderly with dementia-related psychosis	Antipsychotic [Atypical]/mood stabilizer Persistent QTc measurements >500: *D/C ziprasidone.* Evaluate palpitations, syncope. Agents (pimozide) that prolong QT interval are contraindicated. Avoid CNS depressants. *Monitor* BP, pulse, ECG, and for EPS, NMS, and TD; also BMI, FBS, lipids.

Continued

Psychotropic Drugs A – Z (Alphabetical Listing)—cont'd

Generic (Trade)	Dose Range/ Adult Daily Dose	Use/Common Side Effects (CSE)	Geriatric Assessment & Dose Considerations	Classification Assessment Cautions
Zolpidem (Ambien, Ambien CR, Intermezzo) T½ = 2.5–2.6 h Schedule IV Pregnancy category B	Range: 5–10 mg hs Usual: 10 mg po hs; time drowsiness, CR: 12.5 mg po hs Intermezzo sublingual tab: middle-of-night awakening: 1.75/3.5 mg once nightly	Use: Insomnia CSE: Amnesia, cay- diarrhea, physical/ "drugged" feeling, psychological depend- ence (see FDA warn- ing, enc of tab.	In trial ↓ dose; geriatric or hepat- ic disease: Start: 5 mg po hs, may increase to 10 mg; CR: 6.25 mg po hs	Sedative/hypnotic Caution in alcohol abuse and avoid use with CNS depressants. For short-term treat- ment of insomnia; after 2 wk, avoid abrupt withdrawal.

© **ALERT:** Refer to the Physicians' Desk Reference or package insert (prescribing information) for complete and current drug information (dosages, warnings, indications, adverse effects, interactions, etc.) needed to make appropriate choices in the treatment of clients before administering any medications. Although every effort has been made to provide key information about medications and classes of drugs, such information is not and cannot be all-inclusive in a reference of this nature and should not be used for prescribing or administering of medications. Professional judgment, training, supervision, relevant references, and "current" drug information are critical to the appropriate selection, evaluation, and use of drugs, as well as the monitoring and management of clients and their medications.

FDA WARNINGS (2007): The US Food and Drug Administration wants all makers of **antidepressants** to include warnings about increased risk for suicidality in young adults ages 18–24 during initial treatment. The FDA also wants all manufacturers of **sedatives-hypnotics** to warn about possible severe allergic reactions as well as complex sleep-related behaviors, such as sleep-driving. If angioedema develops, seek treatment and do not use drug again. Complete drug monographs located at: http://davisplus.fedavis.com or see inside front cover. Sources: Pedersen Pocket Psych Drugs 2010; Davis's Drug Guide 13th ed. 2012, prescribing information (package inserts).

Crisis/Suicide/Grief/Abuse

Crisis Intervention

Phases

I. Assessment – What caused the crisis, and what are the individual's responses to it?

II. Planning intervention – Explore individual's strengths, weaknesses, support systems, and coping skills in dealing with the crisis.

III. Intervention – Establish relationship, help understand event and explore feelings, and explore alternative coping strategies.

IV. Evaluation/reaffirmation – Evaluate outcomes/Plan for future/Evaluate need for follow-up (Aguilera 1998).

Prevention/Management of Assaultive Behaviors

Assessment of signs of anger is very important in prevention and in intervening before anger escalates to assault/violence.

Early Signs of Anger

■ Muscular tension: clenched fist
■ *Face:* furled brow, glaring eyes, tense mouth, clenched teeth, flushed face
■ *Voice:* raised or lowered

If anger is not identified and recognized at the preassaultive tension stage, it can progress to aggressive behavior.

Anger Management Techniques
- Remain calm
- Help client recognize anger
- Find an outlet: verbal (talking) or physical (exercise)
- Help client accept angry feelings; *not acceptable to act on them*
- Do not touch an angry client
- Medication may be needed

Signs of Anger Escalation
- Verbal/physical threats
- Pacing/appears agitated
- Throwing objects
- Appears suspicious/disproportionate anger
- Acts of violence/hitting

Anger Management Techniques
- Speak in short command sentences: *Joe, calm down.*
- Never allow yourself to be cornered with an angry client; *always have an escape route* (open door behind you)
- *Request assistance of other staff*
- Medication may be needed; *offer voluntarily first*
- Restraints and/or seclusion may be needed *(see Use of Restraints in Basics tab)*
- Continue to *assess/reassess* (ongoing)
- When stabilized, *help client identify early signs/triggers of anger and alternatives* to prevent future anger/escalation

Suicide

Risk Factors Include:
- Mood disorders such as depression and bipolar disorder
- Substance abuse (dual diagnosis)
- Previous suicide attempt
- Loss – marital partner, partner, close relationship, job, health
- Expressed hopelessness or helplessness (does not see a future)
- Impulsivity/aggressiveness
- Family suicides, significant other or friend/peer suicide
- Isolation (lives alone/few friends, support relationships)
- Stressful life event
- Previous or current abuse (emotional/physical/sexual)
- Sexual identity crisis/conflict
- Available lethal method, such as a gun
- Legal issues/incarceration (USPHS, HHS 1999)

Suicide Assessment

- **Hopelessness** – a key element; client is unable to see a future for self in that future.
- **Speaks of suicide (suicidal ideation)** – important to ask client if he/she has thoughts of suicide.
- **Plan** – client is able to provide an exact method for ending life; must take seriously and consider immediately.
- **Giving away possessions** – any actions such as giving away possessions, putting affairs in order (recent will), connecting anew with old friends/family members as a final goodbye.
- **Auditory hallucinations** – commanding client to kill self.
- **Lack of support network** – isolation, few friends or withdrawing from friends/support network.
- **Alcohol/other substance abuse** – drinking alone.
- **Previous suicide attempt or family history of suicide.**
- **Precipitating event** – death of a loved one; loss of a job, especially long-term job; holidays; tragedy; disaster.
- **Media** – suicide of a famous personality or local teenager (Rakel 2000). (See Suicidal Behaviors Questionnaire-R in the Assessment tab.)

CLINICAL PEARL – Do not confuse self-injurious behavior (cutting) with suicide attempts, although those who repeatedly cut themselves to relieve emotional pain could also attempt suicide. "Cutters" may want to stop cutting self but find stopping difficult, as this has become a *pattern of stress reduction.*

Groups at Risk for Suicide

- **Elderly** – especially those who are isolated, widowed; multiple losses, including friends/peers.
- **Males** – especially widowed and without close friends; sole emotional support came from marriage partner who is now deceased.
- **Adolescents and young adults.**
- **Serious/terminal illness** – not all terminally ill clients are suicidal, but should be considered in those who become depressed or hopeless.
- **Mood disorders** – depression and especially bipolar; always observe and assess those receiving treatment for depression, as suicide attempt may take place with improvement of depressive symptoms (client has the energy to commit suicide).
- **Schizophrenia** – newly diagnosed schizophrenics and those with command hallucinations.
- **Substance abusers** – especially with a mental disorder.
- **Stress and loss** – stressful situations and loss can trigger a suicide attempt, especially multiple stressors and losses or a significant loss.

Suicide Interventions

- Effective assessment and knowledge of risk factors
- Observation and safe environment (no "sharps")
- Psychopharmacology, especially the selected serotonin reuptake inhibitors (SSRIs) (children, adolescents, and young adults on SSRIs need to be closely monitored)
- Identification of triggers; educating client as to triggers to seek help early on
- Substance abuse treatment; treatment of pain disorders
- Psychotherapy/cognitive behavioral therapy/electroconvulsive therapy
- Treatment of medical disorders (thyroid/cancer)
- Increased activity if able
- Support network/family involvement
- Involvement in outside activities/avoid isolation – join outside groups, bereavement groups, organizations, care for a pet
- Client and family education

Elder Suicide (see Geriatric tab)

Terrorism/Disasters

With the increase in worldwide terrorism and natural disasters, health-care professionals need to improve their knowledge and awareness of the effects of psychological damage on individuals and communities affected by these disasters. In large-scale disasters:

- Loss can involve individual homes/lives as well as whole communities (neighborhoods).
- Neighbors and friends may be lost as well as reliable and familiar places and supports (neighborhoods, towns, rescue services).

Terrorism and War

- Loss may involve body parts (self-image) and a sense of trust and safety. Previous beliefs may be challenged.
- Individuals may experience shock, disorientation, anger, withdrawal, to name a few feelings/responses.
- The long-term effects on both individuals and future generations cannot be underestimated, and all health-care professionals need to familiarize themselves with disaster and terrorism preparedness.

Military, Families, and PTSD

- In recent wars the use of IEDs and improved immediate medical care has resulted in soldiers surviving and then returning with traumatic brain injuries and the loss of multiple body parts. The Wounded Warrior Project and Joining Forces help injured soldiers (physical/psychological) and their families adjust to a return to society through a variety of programs (www.whitehouse.gov/joiningforces 2013)

- Homelessness has also increased for both men and women soldiers returning home, along with long separations of family members (mothers, fathers, children), resulting in marital/family stress, and repeat tours of duty for men and women with little or no respite in between.

■ Posttraumatic stress has "tripled," since 2001, among military personnel, who are combat exposed (Science News 2008). According to the National Center for PTSD (2012), PTSD occurs in 11%–20% of Iraq and Afghanistan war veterans. (See Posttraumatic Stress Disorder, Substance Use Disorders, and also PTSD Treatments in the Disorders-Interventions tab; see also Mobile Device Apps, PTSD Coach/PE Coach, in the Interventions tab and the Tools tab.)

Death and Dying/Grief

Stages of Death and Dying (Kübler-Ross)

1. *Denial and isolation* – usually a temporary state of being unable to accept the possibility of one's death or that of a loved one.
2. *Anger* – replacement of temporary "stage one" with the reality that death is possible/going to happen. This is the realization that the future (plans/hopes) will have an end; a realization of the finality of the self. May fight/argue with health-care workers/push family/friends away.

Complicated Versus Uncomplicated Grief

Complicated Grief	Uncomplicated Grief
• Excessive in duration (may be delayed reaction or compounded by losses [multiple losses]); usually longer than 3–6 mo	• Follows a major loss
• Disabling symptoms; morbid preoccupation with deceased/physical symptoms	• Depression perceived as normal
• Substance abuse, increased alcohol intake	• Self-esteem intact
• Risk factors: limbo states (missing person), ambivalent relationship, multiple losses; long-term partner (sole dependency); no social network; history of depression	• Guilt specific to lost one (should have telephoned more)
• Suicidal thoughts—may want to join the deceased	• Distress usually resolves within 12 wk (though mourning can continue for 1 or more years)
	• Suicidal thoughts transient or unusual (Shader 2003; mayoclinic.com 2012)

3. *Bargaining* – seeks one last hope or possibility; enters an agreement or pact with God for "one last time or event" to take place before death. *(Let me live to see my grandchild born or my child graduate from college.)*
4. *Depression* – after time, loss, pain, the person realizes that the situation and course of illness will not improve; necessary stage to reach acceptance.
5. *Acceptance* – after working/passing through the previous stages, the person finally accepts what is going to happen; this is not resignation (giving up) or denying and fighting to the very end: it is a stage that allows for peace and dignity (Kübler-Ross 1997).

Victims of Abuse

Cycle of Battering

Phase I. Tension Building – Anger with little provocation; minor battering and excuses. Tension mounts and victim tries to placate. (Victim assumes guilt: I deserve to be abused.)

Phase II. Acute Battering – Most violent, up to 24 hours. Beating may be severe, and victim may provoke to get it over. Minimized by abuser. Help sought by victim if life-threatening or fear for children.

Phase III. Calm, Loving, Respite – Batterer is loving, kind, contrite. Fear of victim leaving. Lesson taught, and now batterer believes victim "understands."

- Victim believes batterer can change, and batterer uses guilt. Victim believes this (calm/loving in phase III) is *what batterer is really like*. Victim hopes the previous phases will not repeat themselves.
- Victim stays because of fear for life (batterer threatens more, and self-esteem lowers), society values marriage, divorce is viewed negatively, financial dependence.

Starts all over again – dangerous, and victim often killed (Walker 1979).
Be aware that victims (of batterers) can be wives, husbands, intimate partners (female/female, male/male, male/female), and pregnant women.

Safety Plan (to Escape Abuser)

- Doors, windows, elevators – *rehearse exit plan.*
- *Have a place to go* – friends, relatives, motel – where you will be and feel safe.
- *Survival kit* – pack and *include money* (cab); change of clothes; identifying info (passports, birth certificate); legal documents, including protection orders; address books; jewelry; important papers.
- Start an *individual checking/savings account.*
- *Always have a safe exit* – do not argue in areas with no exit.
- *Legal rights/domestic hotlines* – know how to contact abuse/legal/domestic hotlines (see Web sites).
- *Review safety plan consistently* (monthly) (Reno 2004).

Signs of Child Abuse (Physical/Sexual)

Physical Abuse	Sexual Abuse
• Pattern of bruises/welts • Burns (e.g., from cigarettes, scalds) • Lesions resembling bites or fingernail marks • Unexplained fractures or dislocations, especially in child younger than 3 y • Areas of baldness from hair pulling • Injuries in various stages of healing • Other injuries or untreated illness, unrelated to present injury • X-rays revealing old fractures	• Signs of genital irritation, such as pain or itching • Bruised or bleeding genitalia • Enlarged vaginal or rectal orifice • Stains and/or blood on underwear • Unusual sexual behavior
Signs Common to Both	
• Signs of "failure to thrive" syndrome • Details of injury changing from person to person • History inconsistent with developmental stages • Parent blaming child or sibling for injury • Parental anger toward child for injury • Parental hostility toward health-care workers	• Exaggeration or absence of emotional response from parent regarding child's injury • Parent not providing child with comfort • Toddler or preschooler not protesting parent's leaving • Child showing preference for health-care worker over parent

Adapted from Myers RNotes 3rd ed., 2010, with permission.

Child Abuser Characteristics
Characteristics associated with those who may be child abusers:

■ In a stressful situation, such as unemployed
■ Poor coping strategies; may be suspicious or lose temper easily
■ Isolated; few support systems or none
■ Do not understand needs of children, basic care, or child development
■ Expect child perfection, and child behavior blown out of proportion (Murray & Zentner 1997)

Incest/Sexual Abuse

Often a father-daughter relationship (biological/stepfather), but can be father-son as well as mother-son. Also applies to any sexual abuse (coach, family friend).

■ Child is made to feel special *(It is our special secret)*; gifts given.
■ Favoritism (becomes intimate friend/sex partner replacing mother/other parent).

- Serious boundary violations and no safe place for child (child's bedroom usually used).
- May be threats if child tells about the sexual activities (Christianson & Blake 1990).

Signs of Incest/Sexual Abuse
- Low self-esteem, sexual acting out, mood changes, sudden poor performance in school
- Parent spends inordinate amount of time with child, especially in room or late at night; very attentive to child
- Child is apprehensive (fearing sexual act/retaliation)
- Alcohol and drugs may be used (Christianson & Blake 1990)

⊚ **ALERT:** All child abuse (physical/sexual/emotional) or child neglect must be reported.

Elder Abuse (see Geriatric tab)

Other Kinds of Abuse

- **Emotional Neglect** — parental/caretaker behaviors include:
  - Ignoring child
  - Ignoring needs (social, educational, developmental)
  - Rebuffing child's attempts at establishing interactions that are meaningful
  - Little to no positive reinforcement (KCAPC 1992)
- **Emotional Injury** – results in serious impairment in child's functioning on all levels:
  - Treatment of child is harsh, with cruel and negative comments, belittling child
  - Child may behave immaturely, with inappropriate behaviors for age
  - Child demonstrates anxiety, tearfulness, sleep disturbances
  - Child shows inappropriate affect, self-destructive behaviors
  - Child may isolate, steal, cheat, as indication of emotional injury (KCAPC 1992)
- **Male Sexual Abuse** – Males are also sexually abused by mothers, fathers, uncles, pedophiles, and others in authority (coach, teacher, minister, priest)
  - Suffer from depression, shame, blame, guilt, and other effects of child sexual abuse
  - Issues related to masculinity, isolation, and struggles with seeking or receiving help
- **Worldwide Child Trafficking** – There are between 12 and 27 million people enslaved in the world today. Fifty percent are women and children and 1.2 million children are trafficked for child labor. An estimated 2 million children are trapped in sexual slavery around the world (www.worldvision.org 2012).
- **Child Pornography** – One of the fastest growing groups in the criminal justice system, likely fueled by Internet access (Hernandez 2009).

Geriatric/Elderly

Geriatric Assessment

Key Points

■ Be mindful that the elderly client may be hard of hearing, but do not assume that all elderly are hard of hearing.
■ Approach and speak to elderly clients as you would any other adult client. It is insulting to speak to the elderly client as if he/she were a child.
■ Eye contact helps instill confidence and, in the presence of impaired hearing, will help the client to understand you better.
■ Be aware that both decreased tactile sensation and ROM are normal changes with aging. Care should be taken to avoid unnecessary discomfort or even injury during a physical exam/assessment.
■ Be aware of generational differences, especially gender differences (i.e., modesty for women, independence for men).
■ Assess for altered mental states.
   ■ **Neurocognitive Disorder:** Cognitive deficits (memory, reasoning, judgment, etc.)
   ■ **Delirium:** Confusion/excitement marked by disorientation to time and place, usually accompanied by illusions and/or hallucinations
   ■ **Depression:** Diminished interest or pleasure in most/all activities

Age-Related Changes and Their Implications

Decreased skin thickness	Elderly clients are more prone to skin breakdown
Decreased skin vascularity	Altered thermoregulation response can put elderly at risk for heatstroke

Continued

Age-Related Changes and Their Implications—cont'd

Loss of subcutaneous tissue	Decreased insulation can put elderly at risk for hypothermia
Decreased aortic elasticity	Produces increased diastolic blood pressure
Calcification of thoracic wall	Obscures heart and lung sounds and displaces apical pulse
Loss of nerve fibers/neurons	The elderly client needs extra time to learn and comprehend and to perform certain tasks
Decreased nerve conduction	Response to pain is altered
Reduced tactile sensation	Puts client at risk for accidental self-injury

From Myers, RNotes, 3rd ed., 2010, with permission

Disorders of Late Life

- **Dementias** – Neurocognitive disorder due to Alzheimer's disease (AD), Lewy body dementia, Vascular neurocognitive disorder, and other neurocognitive disorders. *(See Neurocognitive Disorders in the Disorders-Interventions tab).*
- **Geriatric depression** – Depression in old age is often assumed to be normal; however, depression at any age is not normal and needs to be diagnosed and treated. Factors can include:
  - Physical and cognitive decline
  - Loss of function/self-sufficiency
  - Loss of marriage partner, friends (narrowing support group), isolation
  - The elderly may have many somatic complaints (head hurts, stomach upsets) that mask the depression (Chenitz 1991) *(See Geriatric Depression Scale in Assessment tab)*
- **Pseudodementia** – Cognitive difficulty that is *actually caused by depression but may be mistaken for dementia.*
  - Need to consider and rule out dementia (Mini-Mental State Examination) and actually differentiate from depression (Geriatric Depression Scale)
  - Can be depressed with cognitive deficits as well
- **Late-onset schizophrenia** – Presents later in life, after age 40–60 y.
  - Psychotic episodes (delusions or hallucinations) may be overlooked (schizophrenia is considered to be a young-adult disease)
  - Organic brain disease should be considered as part of the differential diagnosis

Characteristics of Late-Onset Schizophrenia

- *Delusions of persecution* common, hallucinations prominent; "partition" delusion (people/objects pass through barriers and enter home) common; rare in early onset.
- *Sensory deficits* – often auditory/visual impairments
- May have been *previously paranoid, reclusive,* yet functioned otherwise
- *Lives alone/isolated/unmarried*
- *Negative symptoms/thought disorder rare*
- *More common in women* (early onset: equally common) (Lubman & Castle 2002)

Psychotropic Drugs – Geriatric Considerations

(See Drugs A–Z tab for geriatric considerations; and the Elderly and Medications [Drugs/Labs tab].)

Pharmacokinetics in the Elderly

Pharmacokinetics is the way that a drug is absorbed, distributed and used, metabolized, and excreted by the body. Age-related physiological changes affect body systems, altering pharmacokinetics and increasing or altering a drug's effect.

Physiological	Effect on Change	Pharmacokinetics
Absorption	• Decreased intestinal motility	Delayed peak effect
	• Diminished blood flow to the gut	Delayed signs/symptoms of toxic effects
Distribution	• Decreased body water	Increased serum concentration of water-soluble drugs
	• Increased percentage of body fat	Increased half-life of fat-soluble drugs
	• Decreased amount of plasma proteins	Increased amount of active drug
	• Decreased lean body mass	Increased drug concentration
Metabolism	• Decreased blood flow to liver	Decreased rate of drug clearance by liver
	• Diminished liver function	Increased accumulation of some drugs

Continued

Physiological	Effect on Change	Pharmacokinetics
Excretion	• Diminished kidney function	Increased accumulation of drugs excreted by kidney
	• Decreased creatinine clearance	

From Myers, RNotes, 3rd ed., 2010, with permission

Elder Abuse

There are many types of elder abuse, which include:

- *Elder neglect* (lack of care by omission or commission)
- *Psychological* or *emotional abuse* (verbal assaults, insults, threats)
- *Physical* (physical injury, pain, drugs, restraints)
- *Sexual abuse* (nonconsensual sex: rape, sodomy)
- *Financial abuse* (misuse of resources: social security, property)
- *Self-neglect* (elder cannot provide appropriate self-care)

Elder Abuse – Physical Signs
- Hematomas, welts, bites, burns, bruises, and pressure sores
- Fractures (various stages of healing), contractures
- Rashes, fecal impaction
- Weight loss, dehydration, substandard personal hygiene
- Broken dentures, hearing aids, other devices; poor oral hygiene; traumatic alopecia; subconjunctival hemorrhage

Elder Abuse – Behavioral Signs
Caregiver
- Caregiver insistence on being present during entire appointment
- Answers for client
- Caregiver expresses indifference or anger, not offering assistance
- Caregiver does not visit hospitalized client

Elder
- Hesitation to be open, appearing fearful, poor eye contact, ashamed, baby talk
- Paranoia, anxiety, anger, low self-esteem
- *Physical signs:* contractures, inconsistent medication regimen (subthera-peutic levels), malnutrition, poor hygiene, dehydration
- *Financial:* signed over power of attorney (unwillingly), possessions gone, lack of money

Elder Abuse – Medical and Psychiatric History

- Mental health/psychiatric interview
- Assess for depression, anxiety, alcohol (substance) abuse, insomnia
- Functional independence/dependence
- Cognitive impairment (Stiles et al 2002)

@ **ALERT:** All elder abuse must be reported.

Elder Suicide

Warning Signs

- Failed suicide attempt
- Indirect clues – stockpiling medications; purchasing a gun; putting affairs in order; making/changing a will; donating body to science; giving possessions/money away; relationship, social downturns; recent appointment with a physician
- Situational clues – recent move, death of spouse/friend/child
- Symptoms – depression, insomnia, agitation, others

Elder Profile for Potential Suicide

- Male gender
- White
- Divorced or widowed
- Lives alone, isolated, moved recently
- Unemployed, retired
- Poor health, pain, multiple illnesses, terminal
- Depressed, substance abuser, hopeless
- Family history of suicide, depression, substance abuse; early trauma in childhood
- Wish to end hopeless, intolerable situation
- Lethal means: guns, stockpiled sedatives/hypnotics
- Previous attempt
- Not inclined to reach out; often somatic complaints

Suspected Elder Suicidality

Ask direct questions:

- Are you so down you see no point in going on? (If answer is yes, explore further: Tell me more.)
- Have you (ever) thought of killing yourself? (When? What stopped you?)
- How often do you have these thoughts?
- How would you kill yourself? (Lethality plan) (Holkup 2002)

Gather information – keep communication open in a nonjudgmental way; do not minimize or offer advice in this situation. (See Suicidal Behaviors Questionnaire-R [SBQ-R] in the Assessment tab.)

Tools/References/Index

Access more online at DavisPlus:

- DSM-IV-TR and DSM-5 Conversion Guide
- DSM-5 Classification and Codes (including ICD-9-CM and ICD-10-CM Codes)
- Psychotropic Drugs (over 78 complete monographs)
- Psychiatric Assessment Rating Scale Information
- Psychiatric Resources: Organizations/Web sites/Hotlines
- Psychiatric Terminology (Glossary)

Log on to DavisPlus at http://davisplus.FADavis.com Keyword: Pedersen
Clinicians need to sign up as a *student* to access online resources.

Abbreviations

AD Dementia of Alzheimer's type
ADHD Attention deficit hyperactivity disorder
AE Adverse event
AIMS Abnormal Involuntary Movement Scale
BAI Beck Anxiety Inventory
BDI Beck Depression Inventory
BP Blood pressure
BPD Borderline personality disorder
BPH Benign prostatic hypertrophy
CBC Complete blood count
CBT Cognitive behavioral therapy
CHF Congestive heart failure
CK Creatine kinase
CNS Central nervous system
COPD Chronic obstructive pulmonary disease
CT scan Computed tomography scan
CV Cardiovascular
DBT Dialectical behavioral therapy
d/c Discontinue
ECA Epidemiologic Catchment Area Survey
ECG Electrocardiogram
ECT Electroconvulsive therapy
EMDR Eye movement desensitization and reprocessing
EPS Extrapyramidal symptoms
FBS Fasting blood sugar
GABA Gamma-aminobutyric acid
GAD Generalized anxiety disorder
GDS Geriatric Depression Scale
HAM-A Hamilton Anxiety Scale
HAM-D Hamilton Depression Scale
Hx History
LFTs Liver function tests
IM Intramuscular
IV Intravenous

kg Kilogram
L Liter
MAOI Monoamine oxidase inhibitor
MCV Mean corpuscular volume
MDD Major depressive disorder
µg Microgram
mEq Milliequivalent
MH Mental health
mL Milliliter
MMSE Mini-Mental State Exam
MRI Magnetic resonance imaging
MSE Mental Status Exam
NAMI National Association for the Mentally Ill
NCD Neurocognitive disorder
NE Norepinephrine
NMS Neuroleptic malignant syndrome
OCD Obsessive-compulsive disorder
OTC Over the counter
PANSS Positive and Negative Syndrome Scale
PMDD Premenstrual dysphoric disorder
PTSD Posttraumatic stress disorder
SMAST Short Michigan Alcohol Screening Test
SNRI Serotonin-norepinephrine reuptake inhibitor
SSRI Selective serotonin reuptake inhibitor
$T_{1/2}$ Drug's half-life
TCA Tricyclic antidepressant
TFT Thyroid function test
TIA Transient ischemic attack
TPR Temperature, pulse, respiration
UA Urinalysis
UTI Urinary tract infection

Assessment Tools

See Assessment tab for the following tools/rating scales:

- Abnormal Involuntary Movement Scale (AIMS)
- Edinburgh Postnatal Depression Scale (EPDS)
- Geriatric Depression Scale (GDS)
- Hamilton Anxiety Scale (HAM-A)
- Hamilton Depression Scale (HAM-D)
- Ethnocultural Assessment Tool
- The Hoarding Rating Scale
- Mental Status Assessment Tool
- Mood Disorder Questionnaire (MDQ)
- Psychiatric History and Assessment Tool
- Short Michigan Alcohol Screening Test (SMAST)
- Substance History and Assessment
- Suicidal Behaviors Questionnaire (SBQ-R)

Mobile Device Apps

An increasing number of self-rating mood disorder apps are being developed for mobile devices for consumer use. Disclaimers state, rightfully so, that these tools are "for information purposes only" or "not to be used as a diagnostic tool." As long as the consumer understands the tool is not providing an actual diagnosis and seeks professional help when a red flag is raised, the screening may have provided a service. However, without validation of the screening tool, caution is advised and professional evaluation should be advised.

Validated App & Mood/Anxiety Disorder Screening Tool: WhatsMyM3 — My Mood Monitor (M-3 Checklist)

The M-3 Checklist was developed by a team of psychiatrists, family physicians, psychologists, and others and validated in a study performed at the University of North Carolina (Gaynes 2010).

- Three-minute, 27-item rating scale that screens for mood and anxiety disorders, including depression, anxiety, PTSD, and Bipolar that can be used in primary care.
- WhatsMyM3 app for mobile device costs about $0.99.
- Diagnostic accuracy equals current single-disorder screens.
- If there is a red flag for suicide, user can immediately call the National Suicide Prevention Hotline.
- M-3 score of 33 or higher suggests a mood disorder and degree of severity is provided for all four categories, e.g., low, medium, high.
- User can monitor progress (graphically) and treatments at: mymoodmonitor.com (can download app from this website).

DSM-5 CLASSIFICATION AND DISORDERS

Neurodevelopmental Disorders

Intellectual Disabilities
Intellectual Disability (Intellectual Developmental Disorder)
Global Developmental Delay
Unspecified Intellectual Disability (Intellectual Developmental Disorder)

Communication Disorders
Language Disorder
Speech Sound Disorder
Childhood-Onset Fluency Disorder (Stuttering)
Social (Pragmatic) Communication Disorder
Unspecified Communication Disorder

Autism Spectrum Disorder
Autism Spectrum Disorder

Attention-Deficit/Hyperactivity Disorder
Attention-Deficit/Hyperactivity Disorder
Other Specified Attention-Deficit/Hyperactivity Disorder
Unspecified Attention-Deficit/Hyperactivity Disorder

Specific Learning Disorder
Specific Learning Disorder

Motor Disorders
Developmental Coordination Disorder
Stereotypic Movement Disorder

Tic Disorders
Tourette's Disorder
Persistent (Chronic) Motor or Vocal Tic Disorder
Provisional Tic Disorder
Other Specified Tic Disorder
Unspecified Tic Disorder

Other Neurodevelopmental Disorders
Other Specified Neurodevelopmental Disorder
Unspecified Neurodevelopmental Disorder

Schizophrenia Spectrum and Other Psychotic Disorders

Schizotypal (Personality) Disorder
Delusional Disorder
Brief Psychotic Disorder
Schizophreniform Disorder
Schizophrenia
Schizoaffective Disorder
Substance/Medication-Induced Psychotic Disorder
Psychotic Disorder Due to Another Medical Condition
Catatonia Association With Another Mental Disorder (Catatonia Specifier)
Unspecified Catatonia
Catatonic Disorder Due to Another Medical Condition
Other Specified Schizophrenia Spectrum and Other Psychotic Disorder
Unspecified Schizophrenia Spectrum and Other Psychotic Disorder

Bipolar and Related Disorders

Bipolar I Disorder
Bipolar II Disorder
Cyclothymic Disorder
Bipolar and Related Disorder Due to Another Medical Condition
Other Specified Bipolar and Related Disorder
Unspecified Bipolar and Related Disorder

Depressive Disorders

Disruptive Mood Dysregulation Disorder
Major Depressive Disorder
Persistent Depressive Disorder (Dysthymia)
Premenstrual Dysphoric Disorder
Substance/Medication-Induced Depressive Disorder

Depressive Disorder Due to Another Medical Condition
Other Specified Depressive Disorder
Unspecified Depressive Disorder

Anxiety Disorders

Separation Anxiety Disorder
Selective Mutism
Specific Phobia
Social Anxiety Disorder (Social Phobia)
Panic Disorder
Panic Attack Specifier
Agoraphobia
Generalized Anxiety Disorder
Substance/Medication-Induced Anxiety Disorder
Anxiety Disorder Due to Another Medical Condition
Unspecified Anxiety Disorder

Obsessive-Compulsive and Related Disorders

Obsessive-Compulsive Disorder
Body Dysmorphic Disorder
Hoarding Disorder
Trichotillomania (Hair-Pulling Disorder)
Excoriation (Skin-Picking) Disorder
Substance/Medication-Induced Obsessive-Compulsive and Related Disorder
Obsessive-Compulsive and Related Disorder Due to Another Medical Condition
Other Specified Obsessive-Compulsive and Related Disorder
Unspecified Obsessive-Compulsive and Related Disorder

Trauma- and Stressor-Related Disorders

Reactive Attachment Disorder
Disinhibited Social Engagement Disorder
Posttraumatic Stress Disorder (includes Posttraumatic Stress Disorder for Children 6 Years and Younger)
Acute Stress Disorder
Adjustment Disorders
Other Specified Trauma- and Stressor-Related Disorder
Unspecified Trauma- and Stressor-Related Disorder

Dissociative Disorders

Dissociative Identity Disorder
Dissociative Amnesia (specifier: Dissociative fugue)
Depersonalization/Derealization Disorder
Other Specified Dissociative Disorder
Unspecified Dissociative Disorder

Somatic Symptom and Related Disorders

Somatic Symptom Disorder
Illness Anxiety Disorder
Conversion Disorder (Functional Neurological Symptom Disorder)
Psychological Factors Affecting Other Medical Conditions
Factitious Disorder (includes Factitious Disorder Imposed on Self,
Factitious Disorder Imposed on Another)
Other Specified Somatic Symptom and Related Disorder
Unspecified Somatic Symptom and Related Disorder

Feeding and Eating Disorders

Pica
Rumination Disorder
Avoidant/Restrictive Food Intake Disorder
Anorexia Nervosa
Bulimia Nervosa
Binge-Eating Disorder
Other Specified Feeding or Eating Disorder
Unspecified Feeding or Eating Disorder

Elimination Disorders

Enuresis
Encopresis
Other Specified Elimination Disorder
Unspecified Elimination Disorder

Sleep-Wake Disorders

Insomnia Disorder
Hypersomnolence Disorder
Narcolepsy

Breathing-Related Sleep Disorders
Obstructive Sleep Apnea Hypopnea
Central Sleep Apnea
Sleep-Related Hypoventilation
Circadian Rhythm Sleep-Wake Disorders

Parasomnias
Non-Rapid Eye Movement Sleep Arousal Disorders
Nightmare Disorder
Rapid Eye Movement Sleep Behavior Disorder
Restless Legs Syndrome
Substance/Medication-Induced Sleep Disorder
Other Specified Insomnia Disorder
Unspecified Insomnia Disorder
Other Specified Hypersomnolence Disorder
Unspecified Hypersomnolence Disorder
Other Specified Sleep-Wake Disorder
Unspecified Sleep-Wake Disorder

Sexual Dysfunctions

Delayed Ejaculation
Erectile Disorder
Female Orgasmic Disorder
Female Sexual Interest/Arousal Disorder
Genito-Pelvic Pain/Penetration Disorder
Male Hypoactive Sexual Desire Disorder
Premature (Early) Ejaculation
Substance/Medication-Induced Sexual Dysfunction
Other Specified Sexual Dysfunction
Unspecified Sexual Dysfunction

Gender Dysphoria

Gender Dysphoria
  Gender Dysphoria in Children
  Gender Dysphoria in Adolescents and Adults
Other Specified Gender Dysphoria
Unspecified Gender Dysphoria

Disruptive, Impulse-Control, and Conduct Disorders

Oppositional Defiant Disorder
Intermittent Explosive Disorder
Conduct Disorder
Antisocial Personality Disorder
Pyromania
Kleptomania
Other Specified Disruptive, Impulse-Control, and Conduct Disorder
Unspecified Disruptive, Impulse-Control, and Conduct Disorder

Substance-Related and Addictive Disorders

Substance-Related Disorders
Alcohol-Related Disorders
Alcohol Use Disorder
Alcohol Intoxication
Alcohol Withdrawal
Other Alcohol-Induced Disorders
Unspecified Alcohol-Related Disorder

Caffeine-Related Disorders
Caffeine Intoxication
Caffeine Withdrawal
Other Caffeine-Induced Disorders
Unspecified Caffeine-Related Disorder

Cannabis-Related Disorders
Cannabis Use Disorder
Cannabis Intoxication
Cannabis Withdrawal
Other Cannabis-Induced Disorders
Unspecified Cannabis-Related Disorder

Hallucinogen-Related Disorders
Phencyclidine Use Disorder
Other Hallucinogen Use Disorder
Phencyclidine Intoxication
Other Hallucinogen Intoxication
Hallucinogen Persisting Perception Disorder
Other Phencyclidine-Induced Disorders
Other Hallucinogen-Induced Disorders
Unspecified Phencyclidine-Related Disorder
Unspecified Hallucinogen-Related Disorder

Inhalant-Related Disorders
Inhalant Use Disorder
Inhalant Intoxication
Other Inhalant-Induced Disorders
Unspecified Inhalant-Related Disorder

Opioid-Related Disorders
Opioid Use Disorder
Opioid Intoxication
Opioid Withdrawal
Other Opioid-Induced Disorders
Unspecified Opioid-Related Disorder

Sedative-, Hypnotic-, or Anxiolytic-Related Disorders
Sedative, Hypnotic, or Anxiolytic Use Disorder
Sedative, Hypnotic, or Anxiolytic Intoxication
Sedative, Hypnotic, or Anxiolytic Withdrawal
Other Sedative-, Hypnotic-, or Anxiolytic-Induced Disorders
Unspecified Sedative-, Hypnotic-, or Anxiolytic-Related Disorder

Stimulant-Related Disorders
Stimulant Use Disorder (e.g., amphetamine, cocaine)
Stimulant Intoxication
Stimulant Withdrawal
Other Stimulant-Induced Disorders
Unspecified Stimulant-Related Disorder
Amphetamine or other stimulant
Cocaine

Tobacco-Related Disorders
Tobacco Use Disorder
Tobacco Withdrawal
Other Tobacco-Induced Disorders
Unspecified Tobacco-Related Disorder

Other (or Unknown) Substance-Related Disorders
Other (or Unknown) Substance Use Disorder
Other (or Unknown) Substance Intoxication
Other (or Unknown) Substance Withdrawal
Other (or Unknown) Substance-Induced Disorders
Unspecified Other (or Unknown) Substance-Related Disorder

Non-Substance-Related Disorders
Gambling Disorder

Neurocognitive Disorders

Delirium
Other Specified Delirium
Unspecified Delirium

Major and Mild Neurocognitive Disorders

Major or Mild Neurocognitive Disorder Due to Alzheimer's Disease
Probable Major Neurocognitive Disorder Due to Alzheimer's Disease
Possible Major Neurocognitive Disorder Due to Alzheimer's Disease
Mild Neurocognitive Disorder Due to Alzheimer's Disease

Major or Mild Frontotemporal Neurocognitive Disorder
Probable Major Neurocognitive Disorder Due to Frontotemporal Lobar
  Degeneration
Possible Major Neurocognitive Disorder Due to Frontotemporal Lobar
  Degeneration
Mild Neurocognitive Disorder Due to Frontotemporal Lobar Degeneration

Major or Mild Neurocognitive Disorder With Lewy Bodies
Probable Major Neurocognitive Disorder With Lewy Bodies
Possible Major Neurocognitive Disorder With Lewy Bodies
Mild Neurocognitive Disorder With Lewy Bodies

Major or Mild Vascular Neurocognitive Disorder
Probable Major Vascular Neurocognitive Disorder
Possible Major Vascular Neurocognitive Disorder
Mild Vascular Neurocognitive Disorder

Major or Mild Neurocognitive Disorder Due to Traumatic Brain Injury
Major Neurocognitive Disorder Due to Traumatic Brain Injury
Mild Neurocognitive Disorder Due to Traumatic Brain Injury

Substance/Medication-Induced Major or Mild Neurocognitive Disorder

Major or Mild Neurocognitive Disorder Due to HIV Infection
Major Neurocognitive Disorder Due to HIV Infection
Mild Neurocognitive Disorder Due to HIV Infection

Major or Mild Neurocognitive Disorder Due to Prion Disease
Major Neurocognitive Disorder Due to Prion Disease
Mild Neurocognitive Disorder Due to Prion Disease

Major or Mild Neurocognitive Disorder Due to Parkinson's Disease
Major Neurocognitive Disorder Probably Due to Parkinson's Disease
Major Neurocognitive Disorder Possibly Due to Parkinson's Disease
Mild Neurocognitive Disorder Due to Parkinson's Disease

Major or Mild Neurocognitive Disorder Due to Huntington's Disease
Major Neurocognitive Disorder Due to Huntington's Disease
Mild Neurocognitive Disorder Due to Huntington's Disease

Major or Mild Neurocognitive Disorder Due to Another Medical Condition
Major Neurocognitive Disorder Due to Another Medical Condition
Mild Neurocognitive Disorder Due to Another Medical Condition

Major or Mild Neurocognitive Disorder Due to Multiple Etiologies
Major Neurocognitive Disorder Due to Multiple Etiologies
Mild Neurocognitive Disorder Due to Multiple Etiologies

Unspecified Neurocognitive Disorder
Unspecified Neurocognitive Disorder

Personality Disorders

Cluster A Personality Disorders
Paranoid Personality Disorder
Schizoid Personality Disorder
Schizotypal Personality Disorder

Cluster B Personality Disorders
Antisocial Personality Disorder
Borderline Personality Disorder
Histrionic Personality Disorder
Narcissistic Personality Disorder

Cluster C Personality Disorders
Avoidant Personality Disorder
Dependent Personality Disorder
Obsessive-Compulsive Personality Disorder

Other Personality Disorders
Personality Change Due to Another Medical Condition
Other Specified Personality Disorder
Unspecified Personality Disorder

Paraphilic Disorders

Voyeuristic Disorder
Exhibitionistic Disorder
Frotteuristic Disorder
Sexual Masochism Disorder

Sexual Sadism Disorder
Pedophilic Disorder
Fetishistic Disorder
Transvestic Disorder
Other Specified Paraphilic Disorder
Unspecified Paraphilic Disorder

Other Mental Disorders

Other Specified Mental Disorder Due to Another Medical Condition
Unspecified Mental Disorder Due to Another Medical Condition
Other Specified Mental Disorder
Unspecified Mental Disorder

Adapted from the *Diagnostic and Statistical Manual of Mental Disorders*, Fifth
Edition. (Copyright 2013). American Psychiatric Association.

Assigning Nursing Diagnoses (NANDA) to Client Behaviors

Following is a list of client behaviors and the NANDA nursing diagnoses that
correspond to the behaviors and that may be used in planning care for the client
exhibiting the specific behavioral symptoms.

Behaviors	NANDA Nursing Diagnoses
Aggression; hostility	Risk for injury; Risk for other-directed violence
Anorexia or refusal to eat	Imbalanced nutrition: Less than body requirements
Anxious behavior	Anxiety (specify level)
Confusion; memory loss	Confusion, acute/chronic; Disturbed thought processes
Delusions	Disturbed thought processes
Denial of problems	Ineffective denial
Depressed mood or anger turned inward	Dysfunctional grieving

Continued

Behaviors	NANDA Nursing Diagnoses
Detoxification; withdrawal from substances	Risk for injury
Difficulty making important life decision	Decisional conflict (specify)
Difficulty with interpersonal relationships	Impaired social interaction
Disruption in capability to perform usual responsibilities	Ineffective role performance
Dissociative behaviors (depersonalization; derealization)	Disturbed sensory perception (kinesthetic)
Expresses feelings of disgust about body or body part	Disturbed body image
Expresses lack of control over personal situation	Powerlessness
Flashbacks, nightmares, obsession with traumatic experience	Posttrauma syndrome
Hallucinations	Disturbed sensory perception (auditory; visual)
Highly critical of self or others	Low self-esteem (chronic; situational)
HIV-positive; altered immunity	Ineffective protection
Inability to meet basic needs	Self-care deficit (feeding; bathing/hygiene; dressing/grooming; toileting)
Insomnia or hypersomnia	Disturbed sleep pattern
Loose associations or flight of ideas	Impaired verbal communication
Manic hyperactivity	Risk for injury
Manipulative behavior	Ineffective coping
Multiple personalities; gender identity disturbance	Disturbed personal identity
Orgasm, problems with; lack of sexual desire	Sexual dysfunction
Overeating, compulsive	Risk for imbalanced nutrition: More than body requirements
Phobias	Fear
Physical symptoms as coping behavior	Ineffective coping

Continued

Behaviors	NANDA Nursing Diagnoses
Projection of blame; rationalization of failures; denial of personal responsibility	Defensive coping
Ritualistic behaviors	Anxiety (severe); Ineffective coping
Seductive remarks; inappropriate sexual behaviors	Impaired social interaction
Self-mutilative behaviors	Self-mutilation; Risk for self-mutilation
Sexual behaviors (difficulty, limitations, or changes in; reported dissatisfaction)	Ineffective sexuality patterns
Stress from caring for chronically ill person	Caregiver role strain
Stress from locating to new environment	Relocation stress syndrome
Substance use as a coping behavior	Ineffective coping
Substance use (denies use is a problem)	Ineffective denial
Suicidal	Risk for suicide; Risk for self-directed violence
Suspiciousness	Disturbed thought processes; Ineffective coping
Vomiting, excessive, self-induced	Risk for deficient fluid volume
Withdrawn behavior	Social isolation

Used with permission from Townsend, 6e 2014

Pregnancy Categories

Category A
Adequate, well-controlled studies in pregnant women have not shown an increased risk of fetal abnormalities.

Category B
Animal studies have revealed no evidence of harm to the fetus, however, there are no adequate and well-controlled studies in pregnant women.

OR

Animal studies have shown an adverse effect, but adequate and well-controlled studies in pregnant women have failed to demonstrate a risk to the fetus.

Category C
Animal studies have shown an adverse effect and there are no adequate and well-controlled studies in pregnant women.

OR

No animal studies have been conducted and there are no adequate and well-controlled studies in pregnant women.

Category D
Studies, adequate well-controlled or observational, in pregnant women have demonstrated a risk to the fetus. However, the benefits of therapy may outweigh the potential risk.

Category X
Studies, adequate well-controlled or observational, in animals or pregnant women have demonstrated positive evidence of fetal abnormalities. The use of the product is contraindicated in women who are or may become pregnant.

NOTE: The designation UK is used when the pregnancy category is unknown.

References

American Hospital Association. A Patient Care Partnership (2003). Accessed 12/19/10 at: http://www.aha.org/aha/issues/Communicating-With-Patients/pt-care-partnership.html

American Hospital Association. A Patient's Bill of Rights (revised 1992)

American Psychiatric Association. Diagnostic and Statistical Manual of Mental Disorders, 5th ed. Washington, DC: American Psychiatric Association, 2013

American Psychiatric Association. DSM-5 development process includes emphasis on gender and cultural sensitivity: Consideration of how gender, race and ethnicity may affect diagnosis of mental illness. (press release). Feb. 10, 2010

American Psychiatric Association. Position Statement: Principles for Health Care Reform in Psychiatry, 2008

American Psychiatric Association. Rationale to the proposed changes to the personality disorders classification in the DSM-5. Updated May 1, 2012. Accessed 10/14/12 at: DSM5.org

American Psychiatric Nurses Association (APNA). Seclusion and Restraint: Position Statement & Standards of Practice, 2007

Andersson M, Zetterberg H, Minthon L, Blennow K, Londos E. The cognitive profile and CSF biomarkers in dementia with Lewy bodies and Parkinson's disease dementia. Int J Geriatr Psychiatry 2011; Jan 26(1):100–105

Anton RF et al. Comparison of bio-rad %CDT IIA and CD Tect as laboratory markers of heavy alcohol use and their relationships with γ-glutamyl-transferase. Clinical Chemistry 2001; 47:1769–1775

Autonomic nervous system. Table 1: Responses of major organs to autonomic nerve impulses. Update in Anaesthesia 1995; issue 5, article 6. Accessed 1/24/04 at: http://www.nda.ox.ac.uk/wfsa/html/u05/u05_b02.htm

Barr AM et al. The need for speed: An update on methamphetamine addiction. Psychiatr Neurosci 2006; 31(5):301–313

Bateson G. Mind and Nature: A Necessary Unity. London: Wildwood House, 1979

Bateson G. Steps to an Ecology of Mind. London: Paladin, 1973

Bleuler E. Dementia Praecox or the Group of Schizophrenias (Zinkin J, trans.). New York: International University Press, 1911

Bohnen NI, Djang DS et al. Effectiveness and safety of 18F-FDG PET in the evaluation of dementia: A review of the recent literature. J Nucl Med 2012; 53(1):59–71

Boszormenyi-Nagy I, Krasner BR. Between Give and Take: A Clinical Guide to Contextual Therapy. New York: Brunner/Mazel, 1986

Bowen M. Family Therapy in Clinical Practice. New Jersey: Aronson, 1994

Brigham and Women's Hospital. Depression: A Guide to Diagnosis and Treatment. Boston, MA: Brigham and Women's Hospital, 2001:9

Brown AS, Susser ES. Epidemiology of schizophrenia: Findings implicate neurodevelopmental insults early in life. In: Kaufman CA, Gorman JM, eds. Schizophrenia: New Directions for Clinical Research and Treatment. Larchmont, NY: Mary Ann Liebert, Inc., 1996:105–119

Brown GW, Birley JL, Wing JK. Influence of family life on the course of schizophrenic disorders: A replication. Br J Psychiatry 1972; 121(562):241–258

Buse JB et al. A retrospective cohort study of diabetes mellitus and antipsychotic treatment in the United States. J Clin Epidemiol 2003; 56:164–170

Carli V, Durkee T et al. The association between pathological Internet use and comorbid psychopathology: A systematic review. Psychopathology 2012 Jul 31 [ePub]

Cattie JE, Woods SP et al. Elevated neurobehavioral symptoms are associated with everyday functioning problems in chronic methamphetamine users. J Neuropsychiatry Clin Neurosci 2012; 1:24(3):331–339

Child Abuse Prevention Treatment Act, originally enacted in 1974 (PL 93–247), 42 USC 5101 et seq; 42 USC 5116 et seq. Accessed 9/25/04 at: http://www. acf.hhs.gov/programs/cb/laws/capta/

Christianson JR, Blake RH. The grooming process in father-daughter incest. In: Horton A, Johnson BL, Roundy LM, Williams D, eds. The Incest Perpetrator: A Family Member No One Wants to Treat. Newbury Park, CA: Sage, 1990:88–98

Christy A, Handelsman JB, Hanson A, Ochshorn E. Who initiates emergency commitments? Community Ment Health J 2010; Apr 46(2): 188–191

Clinical Key. Psychiatry: schizophrenia. Accessed 12/30/12 at: http://www.clinicalkey.com/topics/psychiatry/schizophrenia

Combs DR, Waguspack J, Chapman D et al. An examination of social cognition, neurocognition, and symptoms as predictors of social functioning in schizophrenia. Schizophr Res 2010; Dec 13 [Epub]

Cruz M, Pincus HA. Research on the influence that communication in psychiatric encounters has on treatment. Psychiatr Serv 2002; 53:1253–1265

Cyberonics (2007). Accessed 10/21/12 at: http://www.VNSTherapy.com

Cycle of Violence. Accessed 10/15/12 at: http://www.ojp.usdoj.gov/ovc/help/cycle.htm

Davies T. Psychosocial factors and relapse of schizophrenia [editorial]. BMJ 1994; 309:353–354

DeAngelis T. Is Internet addiction real? Monitor on Psychology. American Psychological Association 2000; 31: No. 4. Accessed 11/27/2006 at: www.apa.org/monitor/apr00/addiction.html

de Souza SD et al: Hologram QSAR models of 4-[(Diethylamino)methyl]-phenol inhibitors of acetyl/butyrlcholinesterase enzymes as potential anti-Alzheimer agents. Molecules 2012; 17:9529–9539

Delrieu J, Ousset P, Caillaud C et al. Clinical trials in Alzheimer's disease: Immunotherapy approaches. J Neurochem 2012; 120(suppl 1):186–193

Drach LM. Drug treatment of dementia with Lewy bodies and Parkinson's disease dementia–common features and differences. Med Monnatsschr Pharm 2011; 34(2):47–52

DSM 5.org. Accessed multiple times at: http://www.dsm5.org/Pages/Default.aspx

Edmondson OJH, Psychogiou L, Vlachos H et al. Depression in fathers in the postnatal period: Assessment of the Edinburgh Postnatal Depression Scale as a screening measure. J Affect Disord 2010; Sept 125(1-3):365–368

Elbogen EB, Wagner HR et al. Correlates of anger and hostility in Iraq and Afganistan war veterans. Am J Psychiatry 2010; 167(9):1051–1058

Emergency Commitments: Psychiatric emergencies. Accessed 1/24/04 at: http://www.pinofpa.org/resources/fact-12.html

Faraone S. Prevalence of adult ADHD in the US [abstract]. Presented at American Psychiatric Association, May 6, 2004. Accessed 10/21/12 at: http://www.pslgroup.com/dg/2441a2.htm

Ferretti MT et al: Minocycline corrects early, pre-plaque neuroinflammation and inhibits BASE-1 in a transgenic model of Alzheimer's disease-like amyloid pathology. J Neuroinflammation 2012; 2–9:62

Folstein M, Folstein SG, McHugh P. Mini-Mental State, a practical method for grading the cognitive state of patients for the clinician. J Psychiatr Res 1975; 12:189–198

Fox S. DSM-V, Healthcare reform will fuel major changes in addiction psychiatry. Medscape medical news 2010. Accessed 10/21/12 at: http://www.medscape.com/viewarticle/733649

Freeman A et al. Clinical Applications of Cognitive Therapy, 2nd ed. New York: Springer Verlag, 2004

George MS, Lisanby SH, Avery D et al. Daily left prefrontal transcranial magnetic stimulation therapy for major depressive disorder. Arch Gen Psychiatry 2010; 67(5):507–516

Ghaemi SN et al. Antidepressants in bipolar disorder: The case for caution. Bipolar Disord 2003; 5:421–433

Goroll AH, Mulley AG Jr. Primary Care Medicine: Office Evaluation and Management of the Adult Patient, 6th ed. Philadelphia: Lippincott Williams & Wilkins, 2009

Guerry JD, Hastings PD. In search of HPA axis dysregulation in child and adolescent depression. Clin Child Fam Psychol Rev 2011; 14(2):135–160

Guy W, ed. ECDEU Assessment Manual for Psychopharmacology. (DHEW Publ. No. 76–338), rev. ed. Washington, DC: US Department of Health, Education and Welfare, 1976

Health Insurance Portability and Accountability Act (HIPAA). Accessed 10/21/12 at: http://www.ihs.gov/AdminMngrResources/HIPAA/index.cfm

Hernandez AE. Global Symposium: Examining the relationship between online and offline offenses and preventing the sexual exploitation of children, April 5-7, 2009. Accessed Dec 29, 2010 at: http://www.iprc.unc.edu/G8/Hernandez_position_paper_Global_Symposium.pdf

Hirschfeld RM, Williams JB, Spitzer RL et al. Development and validation of a screening instrument for bipolar spectrum disorder: The Mood Disorder Questionnaire. Am J Psychiatry 2000; 157:1873–1875

Hirschfeld RMA, Holzer C, Calabrese JR, Weissman M, Reed M, Davies M, Frye MA, Keck P et al. Validity of the Mood Disorder Questionnaire: A general population study. Am J Psychiatry 2003; 160:178–180

Holkup P. Evidence-based protocol: Elderly suicide: Secondary prevention. Iowa City: University of Iowa Gerontological Nursing Interventions Research Center, Research Dissemination Core, June 2002:56

Hunt M. The Story of Psychology. New York: Anchor Books, 2007

International Society of Psychiatric–Mental Health Nurses (ISPN). ISPN Position statement on the use of seclusion and restraint (November 1999). Accessed 10/21/12 at: http://www.ispn-psych.org

Jahoda M. Current Concepts of Positive Mental Health. New York: Basic Books, 1958

Javidi H, Yadollahie M. Post-traumatic stress disorder. Int J Occup Environ Med 2012; 3(1):2–9

Joint Commission on Accreditation of Healthcare Organizations (JCAHO 2005). Restraint and Seclusion, revised April 1, 2005. Accessed 11/25/06 at: http://www.jcaho.org/

Kansas Child Abuse Prevention Council (KCAPC). A Guide about Child Abuse and Neglect. Wichita, KS: National Committee for Prevention of Child Abuse and Parents Anonymous, 1992

Keck PE Jr. Evaluating treatment decisions in bipolar depression. MedScape July 30, 2003. Accessed 10/21/12 at: http:www. medscape.com/viewprogram/ 2571

Kerr ME, Bowen M. Family Evaluation. New York: WW Norton, 1988

Kim H, Chang M et al. Predictors of caregiver burden in caregivers of individuals with dementia. J Adv Nurs 2012; 68(4):846–855

Kübler-Ross E. On Death and Dying. New York: Touchstone, 1997

Kukull WA, Bowen JD. Dementia epidemiology. Med Clin North Am 2002; 86:3

Lewis Fernandez R, Hinton DE et al. Culture and the anxiety disorders: Recommendations for DSM-V (review). Depress Anxiety 2010; 27(2):212–229

Linehan MM. Cognitive-Behavioral Treatment of Borderline Personality Disorder. New York: Guilford Press, 1993

Lippitt R, White RK. An experimental study of leadership and group life. In Maccoby EE, Newcomb TM, Hartley EL, eds. Readings in Social Psychology, 3rd ed. New York: Holt Rinehart & Winston, 1958

Lubman DI, Castle DJ. Late onset schizophrenia: Make the right diagnosis when psychosis emerges after age 60. Curr Psychiatry Online 2002; 1(12).

Major Theories of Family Therapy. Accessed 10/21/12 at: http://www.goldentriadfilms.com/films/theory.htm

Manos PJ. 10-point clock test screens for cognitive impairment in clinic and hospital settings. Psychiatric Times 1998; 15(10). Accessed 10/15/12 at: http://www.psychiatrictimes.com/p981049.html

Mataix-Cols D, Frost RO et al. Hoarding disorder: A new diagnosis for the DSM-V (Review). Depress Anxiety 2010; 27:556–572

Mayo Clinic. Mayo Clinic study using structural MRI may help accurately diagnose dementia patients (July 11, 2009). Accessed 10/21/12 at: http://www.mayoclinic.org/news2009-rst/5348.html

McGoldrick M, Giordano J, Garcia-Preto N. Ethnicity and Family Therapy, 3rd ed. New York: Guilford Press, 2005

Melrose S. Paternal postpartum depression: How can nurses begin to help? Contemp Nurse 2010 Feb-Mar; 34(2):199–210

Meltzer HY, Baldessarini RJ. Reducing the risk for suicide in schizophrenia and affective disorders: Academic highlights. J Clin Psychiatry 2003; 64:9

Mentalhealthcarereform.org. Accessed 10/19/12

Mini-Mental State Examination form. Available from Psychological Assessment Resources, Inc., 16204 North Florida Ave, Lutz, Florida (see http://www.parinc.com/index.cfm)

M'Naughton Rule. Psychiatric News 2002; 37(8)

Monroe-DeVita M, Morse G, Bond GR. Program fidelity and beyond: Multiple strategies and criteria for ensuring quality of assertive community treatment. Psychiatr Serv 2012; 63(8):743–750

Murray RB, Zentner JP. Health Assessment and Promotion Strategies through the Life Span, 6th ed. Stamford, CT: Appleton & Lange, 1997

Myers E. RNotes: Nurses Clinical Pocket Guide, 3rd ed. Philadelphia: FA Davis, 2010

Nagy Ledger of Merits. Accessed 8/2/04 at: http://www. behavenet.com/capsules/treatment/famsys/ldgermrts.htm

National Institute on Alcohol Abuse and Alcoholism (NIAAA). Alcohol Screening and Brief Intervention. Accessed 10/15/12 at: http://pubs.niaaa.nih.gov/publications/Practitioner/pocketguide/pocket_guide.htm. Pocket Guide to Alcohol Screening and Brief Intervention

National Institutes of Health (US). Grady C. Informed consent: The ideal and the reality, Session 5. Aired November 9, 2005; permanent link: http://videocast.nih.gov/Summary.asp?File=12895. Accessed 12/19/10

National Institute of Mental Health (NIMH). The numbers count: Mental disorders in America. Accessed 12/26/10 at: http://www.nimh.nih.gov/health/publications/the-numbers-count-mental-disorders-in-america/index.shtml

Neilsen J, Skadhede S, Correll CU. Antipsychotics associated with the development of type 2 diabetes in antipsychotic-naïve schizophrenia patients. Neuropsychopharmacology 2010; 35: Aug 2010

Nelson JC, Mankoski R, Baker RA. Effects of aripiprazole adjunctive to standard antidepressant treatment on the core symptoms of depression: A post-hoc, pooled analysis of two large, placebo-controlled studies. 2010-01, J Affect Disord 120(1-3):133–140.

Nemeroff CB et al. VNS therapy in treatment-resistant depression: Clinical evidence and putative neurobiological mechanisms. Neuropsychopharmacology 2006; 31:1345–1355

Ng BD, Wiemer-Hastings P. Addiction to the Internet and online gaming. Cyberpsychol Behav 2005; 8:110–113

Paquette M. Managing anger effectively. Accessed 8/2/04 at: http://www.nurseweek.com/ce/ce290a.html

Patient's Bill of Rights: American Hospital Association. Accessed 1/18/04 at: http://joann980.tripod.com/myhomeontheweb/id20.html

Pedersen D. Pocket Psych Drugs: Point of care clinical guide. Philadelphia: FA Davis, 2010

Peplau H. A working definition of anxiety. In: Bird S, Marshall M, eds. Some Clinical Approaches to Psychiatric Nursing. New York: Macmillan, 1963

Peplau HE. Interpersonal Relations in Nursing. New York: Springer, 1992

Purnell LD. Guide to Culturally Competent Health Care, 2nd ed. Philadelphia: FA Davis, 2009

Purnell LD, Paulanka BJ. Transcultural Health Care: A Culturally Competent Approach, 4th ed. Philadelphia: FA Davis 2013

Quality and Safety Education for Nurses (QSEN). Accessed 10/21/12 at: http://www.qsen.org

Rachid F, Bertschy G. Safety and efficacy of repetitive transcranial magnetic stimulation in the treatment of depression: A critical appraisal of the last 10 years. Neurophysiol Clin 2006; 36:157–183

Rakel R. Saunders Manual of Medical Practice, 2nd ed. Philadelphia: WB Saunders, 2000

Reiger DA et al. Comorbidity of mental disorders with alcohol and other drug abuse. JAMA 1990; 246:2511–2518

Reno J. Domestic Violence Awareness. Office of the Attorney General. Accessed 9/25/04 at: http://www.ojp.usdoj.gov/ovc/help/cycle.htm (last updated 4/19/2001)

Rolinski M et al: Cholinesterase inhibitors for dementia with Lewy bodies, Parkinson's disease dementia, and cognitive impairment in Parkinson's disease. Cochrane Database Syst Rev 2012; (3):CD006504

Rosner S, Hackl-Herrwerth A, Leucht S, Vecchi S, Sisurapanont M, Soyka M. Opioid antagonists for alcohol dependence. Cochrane Database Syst Rev. 2010; Dec 8:12

Satcher D. Mental Health: A Report of the Surgeon General. Rockville, MD: US Department of Health and Human Services, Substance Abuse and Mental Health Services Administration, Center for Mental Health Services, National Institutes of Health, National Institute of Mental Health, 1999. Accessed 1/19/04 at: http://www.surgeongeneral.gov/library/mentalhealth/home.html

Scanlon VC, Sanders T. Essentials of Anatomy and Physiology, 6th ed. Philadelphia: FA Davis, 2011

Schloendorff v. Society of New York Hospital, 105 NE 92 (NY 1914)

Schwarz E, Izmailov R, Spain M. Validation of a blood-based laboratory test to aid in the confirmation of a diagnosis of schizophrenia. Biomarker Insights 2010; 5:39–47

Science News (Jan 17, 2008). Post traumatic stress tripled among combat-exposed military personnel. Accessed 1/3/11 at: http://www.sciencedaily.com/releases/2008/01/080116193412.htm

Segal ZV, Bieling P, Young T et al. Antidepressant monotherapy vs sequential pharmacotherapy and mindfulness-based cognitive therapy, or placebo, for relapse prophylaxis in recurrent depression. Arch Gen Psychiartry 2010; 67(12):1256–1264

Selye H. The Stress of Life. New York: McGraw-Hill, 1976

Selzer ML, Vinokur A, van Rooijen L. A self-administered Short Michigan Alcoholism Screening Test (SMAST). J Stud Alcohol 1975; 36:117–126

Shapiro F. Eye Movement Desensitization and Reprocessing: Basic Principles, Protocols, and Procedures, 2nd ed. New York: Guilford Press, 2001

Sheikh JI, Yesavage JA. Geriatric Depression Scale (GDS): Recent evidence and development of a shorter version. In: Brink TL, ed. Clinical Gerontology: A Guide to Assessment and Intervention. New York: Haworth Press, 1986:165–173

Skinner K. The therapeutic milieu: Making it work. J Psychiatr Nursing Mental Health Serv 1979; 17:38–44

Smith M, Hopkins D, Peveler RC et al. First- v. second-generation antipsychotics and risk for diabetes in schizophrenia: Systematic review and meta-analysis. Br J Psychiatry 2008; Jun 192(6):406–411

Stiles MM, Koren C, Walsh K. Identifying elder abuse in the primary care setting. Clin Geriatr 2002; 10. Accessed 8/7/04 at: http://www.mmhc.com

Suicide Risk Factors. Accessed 8/7/04 at: http://www.infoline.org/crisis/ risk.asp

Susser E, Schwartz S, Morabia A, Bromet, E. Psychiatric Epidemiology: Searching for the Causes of Mental Disorders. New York: Oxford University Press, 2006

Tai B, Blaine J. Naltrexone: An Antagonist Therapy for Heroin Addiction. Presented at the National Institute on Drug Abuse, November 12–13, 1997. Accessed 7/3/2004 at: http://www.nida.nih.gov/MeetSum/naltrexone.html

Tarasoff v. Regents of University of California (17 Cal. 3d 425 – July 1, 1976. S. F. No. 23042)

Timpano KR, Exner C et al. The epidemiology of the proposed DSM-5 hoarding disorder: Exploration of the acquisition specifier, associated features, and distress. J Clin Psychiatry 2011; 72(6):780–786

Tolin DE, Stevens MC, Villavicencio AL et al. Neural mechanisms of decision making in hoarding disorder. Arch Gen Psychiatry 2012; 69(8):832–841

Townsend MC. Essentials of Psychiatric Mental Health Nursing: Concepts of Care in Evidence Based Practice, 6th ed. Philadelphia: FA Davis, 2014

Townsend MC. Psychiatric Mental Health Nursing: Concepts of Care in Evidence-Based Practice, 7th ed. Philadelphia: FA Davis, 2012

Travelbee J. Interpersonal Aspects of Nursing. Philadelphia: FA Davis, 1971

Tucker K. Milan Approach to Family Therapy: A Critique. Accessed 10/21/12 at: http://www.priory.com/psych/milan.htm

US Department of Health and Human Services: HIPAA. Accessed 10/21/12

US Public Health Services (USPHS). The Surgeon General's Call to Action to Prevent Suicide. Washington, DC: US Department of Health and Human Services, 1999. Accessed 1/18/04 at: http://www.surgeongeneral. gov/library/calltoaction/calltoaction.htm

Vallerand AH, Sanoski CA. Davis's Drug Guide for Nurses, 13th ed. Philadelphia: FA Davis, 2012

Van der Kolk BA. Trauma and memory. In: Van der Kolk BA, McFarlane AC, Weisaeth L. Traumatic Stress. New York: Guilford Press, 1996

Van Leeuwen AM, Poelhuis-Leth DJ, Bladh ML. Davis's Comprehensive Handbook of Laboratory and Diagnostic Tests with Nursing Implications, 5th ed. Philadelphia: FA Davis, 2013

VeriPsych Biomarker Blood Test. Accessed 12/24/10 at: http://www.veripsych.com/physician-faq

Vernurm P, Jack CR Jr. Role of structural MRI in Alzheimer's disease. Alzheimer's Res Ther 2010; Aug 31 (4):23

Virginia S. In Allyn & Bacon Family Therapy Web Site. Accessed 8/2/04 at: http://www.abacon.com/famtherapy/satir.html

Walker LE. The Battered Woman. New York: Harper & Row, 1979

Warner R. Does the scientific evidence support the recovery model? The Psychiatrist Online 2010; 34:3–5

WebMD Video: Caregiver Stress. Accessed 12/20/10 at: http://www.webmd.com/video/caregiving-stress

World Health Organization (WHO) (1975, 2002). Sexual Health and Sex. Accessed 10/21/12 at: http://www.who.int/reproductive-health/gender/sexual_health.html

Yalom ID, Leszcz M. The Theory and Practice of Group Psychotherapy, 5th ed. New York: Perseus Books, 2005

Yesavage JA et al. Development and validation of a geriatric depression screening scale: A preliminary report. J Psychiatr Res 1983; 17:37–49

Yidiz SH, Ozdemir EM et al. Association of Alzheimer's disease with APOE and IL-1 α gene polymorphisms. Am J Alzheimers Dis Other Dem 2012 Oct 4 [ePub]

Zeanah CH, Gleason MM. Reactive Attachment Disorder: A review for DSM-V. Accessed 10/15/12 at: DSM5.org

Credits

Dosage and drug data in Psychotropic Drug Tab from Vallerand AH, Sanoski CA. Davis's Drug Guide for Nurses, 13th ed. Philadelphia: FA Davis, 2012, and Pedersen: Pocket Psych Drugs, Philadelphia, FA Davis, 2010, with permission, as well as drug package insert prescribing information.

Index